Welcome to **_"The Galveston Diet Cookbook for Menopause: 110+ Recipes Nourishing for Balanced Hormones"._** This book is your comprehensive guide to navigating the unique nutritional needs of menopause with the Galveston Diet, a program specifically designed to support women during this transformative phase of life.

Menopause marks a significant transition, bringing with it a host of changes that can affect your overall well-being. Hormonal fluctuations can lead to symptoms like hot flashes, weight gain, mood swings, and fatigue. While these changes are natural, the right nutrition can make a profound difference in how you feel and function during this time.

The Galveston Diet, is not just another fad diet; it's a scientifically-backed approach that emphasizes anti-inflammatory foods, intermittent fasting, and a low-carb lifestyle. This diet focuses on nourishing your body with wholesome, nutrient-dense foods that can help balance hormones, reduce inflammation, and promote a healthy weight.

In this cookbook, you'll find over 110 delicious and easy-to-prepare recipes designed to support your health and well-being during menopause. These recipes are crafted to provide the essential nutrients your body needs, while also being mindful of the common challenges faced during menopause.

Here's what you can expect to find in this book:

Chapter Highlights:

- **_Breakfasts to Boost Your Morning:_** Start your day with nutrient-rich breakfasts that stabilize blood sugar levels and provide sustained energy.

- **_Lunches to Keep You Energized_**: Satisfying and balanced lunch options that are perfect for on-the-go or a leisurely meal at home.

- **_Dinners for Hormonal Harmony:_** Flavorful and nourishing dinner recipes that support a restful night's sleep and promote hormonal balance.

- **_Snacks and Smoothies:_** Healthy snacks and smoothies that curb cravings and provide a quick nutrient boost.

- **_Desserts with a Purpose:_** Indulgent yet healthy desserts that satisfy your sweet tooth without disrupting your hormonal balance.

Benefits of the Galveston Diet for Menopause:

- ***Hormonal Balance:*** Foods rich in phytoestrogens and other hormone-balancing nutrients.

- ***Reduced Inflammation:*** Anti-inflammatory ingredients to help reduce menopausal symptoms.

- ***Weight Management:*** Low-carb and nutrient-dense recipes to support a healthy weight.

- ***Improved Energy Levels:*** Meals designed to stabilize blood sugar and provide long-lasting energy.

- ***Enhanced Mood:*** Nutrients that support mental well-being and help combat mood swings.

As you embark on this culinary journey, remember that nourishing your body is a powerful way to embrace and celebrate this new chapter of your life. Each recipe is a step towards a healthier, more vibrant you.

So, let's dive in and discover how delicious and empowering the Galveston Diet can be. Here's to balanced hormones, reduced inflammation, and a radiant, thriving life during menopause!

Warm regards,

1. Quinoa•Stuffed Bell Peppers

Ingredient:

• 4 bell peppers (any color)
• 1 cup cooked quinoa
• 1/2 cup diced onion
• 1 clove garlic, minced
• 1/2 cup diced tomatoes
• 1/4 cup crumbled feta cheese
• 2 tbsp chopped fresh parsley
• 1 tsp olive oil
• Salt and pepper to taste

Instructions:

1. Preheat oven to 375°F.

2. Cut the tops off the bell peppers and remove the seeds and membranes. Place the peppers in a baking dish.

3. In a medium bowl, combine the cooked quinoa, onion, garlic, tomatoes, feta cheese, parsley, olive oil, salt, and pepper. Mix well.

4. Stuff the quinoa mixture into the hollowed•out bell peppers.

5. Bake for 25•30 minutes, or until the peppers are tender and the filling is hot.

6. Serve warm.

This recipe is suitable for menopause as it is:
• High in fiber and protein from the quinoa
• Contains vegetables (bell peppers and tomatoes) that provide important nutrients
• Uses healthy fats from the olive oil
• Includes calcium•rich feta cheese
• Avoids processed or high•sodium ingredients

The Galveston Diet recommends focusing on whole, nutrient•dense foods like these to help manage menopausal symptoms.

2. Salmon with Lemon Dill Sauce

Ingredient:

• 4 salmon fillets (about 6 oz each)
• 2 tbsp olive oil
• Salt and pepper to taste

For the Lemon Dill Sauce:
• 1/2 cup sour cream
• 2 tbsp fresh lemon juice
• 1 tbsp chopped fresh dill
• 1 tsp grated lemon zest
• 1 garlic clove, minced
• Salt and pepper to taste

Instructions:

1. Preheat oven to 400°F. Line a baking sheet with parchment paper.

2. Place the salmon fillets on the prepared baking sheet. Drizzle with olive oil and season with salt and pepper.

3. Bake for 12•15 minutes, or until the salmon is cooked through and flakes easily with a fork.

4. Meanwhile, make the lemon dill sauce. In a small bowl, whisk together the sour cream, lemon juice, dill, lemon zest, and garlic. Season with salt and pepper to taste.

5. Serve the baked salmon fillets warm, with the lemon dill sauce spooned over the top.

3. Chia Seed Pudding

Ingredient:

• 1/4 cup chia seeds
• 1 cup unsweetened almond milk
• 1 tbsp maple syrup (or honey)
• 1 tsp vanilla extract
• 1/4 tsp ground cinnamon
• Pinch of sea salt

Instructions:

1. In a medium bowl, whisk together the chia seeds, almond milk, maple syrup, vanilla, cinnamon, and salt until well combined.

2. Cover and refrigerate for at least 2 hours, or overnight, stirring occasionally, until thickened to a pudding•like consistency.

3. Serve chilled, topped with fresh berries, nuts, or additional cinnamon if desired.

Why this recipe is suitable for menopause:

• Chia seeds are a great source of fiber, protein, and omega•3 fatty acids, which can help support hormone balance and overall health during menopause.

• Almond milk is a dairy•free, low•calorie option that is gentle on the digestive system.

• Maple syrup or honey provide a touch of natural sweetness without spiking blood sugar levels.

• Cinnamon is a warming spice that can help regulate blood sugar and reduce inflammation.

This chia seed pudding makes for a satisfying, nutrient•dense snack or breakfast that can help nourish your body during the menopausal transition. Enjoy!

4. Turkey and Vegetable Stir•Fry

Ingredient:

• 1 lb ground turkey
• 2 tbsp sesame oil
• 3 cloves garlic, minced
• 1 tbsp grated fresh ginger
• 1 red bell pepper, sliced
• 1 cup broccoli florets
• 1 cup sliced mushrooms
• 1 cup snow peas or snap peas
• 2 tbsp low•sodium soy sauce or tamari
• 1 tbsp rice vinegar
• 1 tsp sesame seeds (optional)
• Salt and pepper to taste

Instructions:

1. In a large skillet or wok, heat the sesame oil over medium•high heat.

2. Add the ground turkey and cook, breaking it up with a wooden spoon, until browned and cooked through, about 5•7 minutes.

3. Add the garlic and ginger and cook for 1 minute, until fragrant.

4. Add the bell pepper, broccoli, mushrooms, and snow peas. Stir•fry for 3•5 minutes, until the vegetables are tender•crisp.

5. Stir in the soy sauce and rice vinegar. Season with salt and pepper to taste. Serve the turkey and vegetable stir•fry hot, garnished with sesame seeds if desired.

Why this recipe is suitable for menopause:

• Ground turkey is a lean protein source that is gentle on the digestive system.
• The variety of vegetables provides a range of essential vitamins, minerals, and antioxidants to support overall health during menopause.
• Ginger and soy sauce are anti•inflammatory ingredients that can help manage menopausal symptoms.
• The dish is low in added sugars and carbohydrates, which can help maintain stable blood sugar levels.

This turkey and vegetable stir•fry makes for a quick, nutritious, and flavorful meal that can be enjoyed during the menopausal transition.

5. Roasted Sweet Potato and Kale Salad

Ingredient:

- 2 medium sweet potatoes, peeled and cubed
- 2 tbsp olive oil
- Salt and pepper to taste
- 4 cups chopped kale, stems removed
- 1/4 cup toasted pumpkin seeds
- 2 tbsp crumbled feta cheese (optional)

For the Dressing:
- 2 tbsp olive oil
- 1 tbsp apple cider vinegar
- 1 tsp Dijon mustard
- 1 tsp honey
- 1 garlic clove, minced
- Salt and pepper to taste

Instructions:

1. Preheat the oven to 400°F. Toss the cubed sweet potatoes with 2 tbsp olive oil and season with salt and pepper. Spread on a baking sheet and roast for 20•25 minutes, until tender and lightly browned.

2. In a large bowl, combine the roasted sweet potatoes, chopped kale, toasted pumpkin seeds, and feta cheese (if using).

3. In a small bowl, whisk together the ingredients for the dressing: olive oil, apple cider vinegar, Dijon mustard, honey, garlic, salt, and pepper.

4. Drizzle the dressing over the salad and toss gently to coat.

5. Serve the Roasted Sweet Potato and Kale Salad warm or at room temperature.

This salad is a great source of fiber, vitamins, and antioxidants. The roasted sweet potatoes provide complex carbohydrates, while the kale and pumpkin seeds offer a boost of protein and healthy fats. The tangy•sweet dressing ties all the flavors together for a delicious and nutritious meal.

6. Coconut Curry Chicken

Ingredient:

- 1 tsp ground coriander
- 1 cup full•fat coconut milk
- 1 cup low•sodium chicken broth
- 1 cup chopped cauliflower florets
- 1 cup chopped broccoli florets
- 1 cup chopped spinach or kale
- Salt and pepper to taste
- Chopped cilantro for garnish (optional)

- 1 lb boneless, skinless chicken breasts, cut into 1•inch pieces
- 1 tbsp coconut oil
- 1 onion, diced
- 3 cloves garlic, minced
- 1 tbsp grated fresh ginger
- 2 tsp curry powder
- 1 tsp ground turmeric
- 1 tsp ground cumin

Instructions:

1. In a large skillet or wok, heat the coconut oil over medium•high heat. Add the chicken and cook, stirring occasionally, until lightly browned, about 5 minutes.

2. Add the onion, garlic, and ginger to the skillet. Cook for 2•3 minutes, until fragrant.

3. Stir in the curry powder, turmeric, cumin, and coriander. Cook for 1 minute to toast the spices.

4. Pour in the coconut milk and chicken broth. Bring the mixture to a simmer and add the cauliflower and broccoli. Cook for 5•7 minutes, until the vegetables are tender.

5. Stir in the spinach or kale and cook for 2•3 minutes, until the greens are wilted. Season the coconut curry chicken with salt and pepper to taste. Serve the curry hot, garnished with chopped cilantro if desired. Enjoy!

Why this recipe is suitable for menopause:

- Chicken is a lean protein source that is easy to digest.
- Coconut milk provides healthy fats to support hormone balance.
- The variety of vegetables offers a range of vitamins, minerals, and antioxidants.
- Spices like turmeric, ginger, and coriander have anti•inflammatory properties that can help manage menopausal symptoms.
- The dish is low in added sugars and carbohydrates, which can help maintain stable blood sugar levels.

This coconut curry chicken is a flavorful, nourishing meal that can be enjoyed during the menopausal transition.

7. Mango Avocado Salsa

Ingredient:

• 1 ripe mango, diced
• 1 ripe avocado, diced
• 1/2 red onion, finely chopped
• 1 jalapeño, seeded and finely chopped (optional)
• 1/4 cup chopped fresh cilantro
• 2 tbsp fresh lime juice
• 1 tbsp olive oil
• Salt and pepper to taste

Instructions:

1. In a medium bowl, gently combine the diced mango, avocado, red onion, jalapeño (if using), and cilantro.

2. Drizzle the lime juice and olive oil over the salsa and toss gently to coat.

3. Season with salt and pepper to taste.

4. Cover and refrigerate for at least 30 minutes to allow the flavors to meld.

5. Serve the mango avocado salsa as a dip with baked tortilla chips, or use it as a topping for grilled fish, chicken, or tacos.

Why this recipe is suitable for menopause:

• Mangoes are a good source of vitamins C and A, which can help support immune function and skin health during menopause.
• Avocados are rich in healthy monounsaturated fats, which can help regulate hormone levels and reduce inflammation.
• The combination of mango, avocado, and lime juice provides a refreshing, antioxidant•rich salsa that can help manage menopausal symptoms.
• The optional jalapeño adds a touch of heat, which can help boost metabolism and circulation.
• This salsa is low in added sugars and carbohydrates, making it a suitable snack or condiment during the menopausal transition.

This mango avocado salsa is a versatile, nutrient•dense addition to your menopausal diet. Enjoy it as a dip, topping, or side dish for a healthy and flavorful boost.

8. Lentil Soup

Ingredient:

- 1 tbsp olive oil
- 1 onion, diced
- 3 cloves garlic, minced
- 2 carrots, peeled and diced
- Salt and pepper to taste
- Chopped parsley for garnish (optional)
- 2 celery stalks, diced
- 1 cup dried brown or green lentils, rinsed
- 4 cups low•sodium vegetable or chicken broth
- 1 (14.5 oz) can diced tomatoes
- 2 tsp ground cumin
- 1 tsp dried thyme
- 1 bay leaf

Instructions:

1. In a large pot or Dutch oven, heat the olive oil over medium heat. Add the onion and sauté for 3•4 minutes until translucent.

2. Add the garlic, carrots, and celery. Cook for an additional 2•3 minutes, stirring frequently, until the vegetables are slightly softened.

3. Stir in the lentils, broth, diced tomatoes, cumin, thyme, and bay leaf. Bring the soup to a boil.

4. Reduce the heat to low, cover, and simmer for 20•25 minutes, or until the lentils are tender. Remove the bay leaf. Season the lentil soup with salt and pepper to taste. Serve the lentil soup hot, garnished with chopped parsley if desired.

Why this recipe is suitable for menopause:

- Lentils are a great source of plant•based protein, fiber, and complex carbohydrates, which can help support overall health during menopause.
- The vegetables, such as carrots, celery, and onions, provide a variety of vitamins, minerals, and antioxidants to help manage menopausal symptoms.
- Cumin and thyme are spices with anti•inflammatory properties that can help reduce inflammation and improve digestion.
- This soup is low in added sugars and high in fiber, making it a suitable option for maintaining stable blood sugar levels during the menopausal transition.

The Lentil Soup is a nourishing, comforting, and easy•to•prepare meal that can be enjoyed as part of a balanced menopausal diet. Enjoy it as a main course or a side dish to support your overall health and well•being.

9. Greek Yogurt Parfait

Ingredient:

- 1 cup plain Greek yogurt
- 1/2 cup fresh berries (such as blueberries, raspberries, or strawberries)
- 2 tbsp chopped walnuts or almonds
- 1 tbsp unsweetened shredded coconut (optional)
- 1 tsp honey or maple syrup (optional)

Instructions:

1. In a parfait glass or small bowl, layer the Greek yogurt, fresh berries, and chopped nuts.

2. If desired, sprinkle the shredded coconut over the top.

3. Drizzle a small amount of honey or maple syrup over the parfait, if using.

4. Serve chilled or at room temperature.

Why this recipe is suitable for menopause:

- Greek yogurt is a great source of protein, which can help support muscle mass and bone health during menopause.

- Berries are rich in antioxidants and can help reduce inflammation, which is often a concern during the menopausal transition.

- Nuts, such as walnuts or almonds, provide healthy fats and fiber to help regulate blood sugar levels and support hormone balance.

- Coconut adds a touch of healthy fat and flavor, while the optional honey or maple syrup provides a small amount of natural sweetness.

- This parfait is low in added sugars and carbohydrates, making it a suitable snack or dessert option for managing menopausal symptoms.

The Greek Yogurt Parfait is a simple, yet nutrient•dense treat that can be enjoyed as part of a balanced menopausal diet. The combination of protein, fiber, and antioxidants makes it a great choice to support overall health and well•being during this transitional time.

10. Baked Apples with Cinnamon

Ingredient:

• 4 medium•sized apples (such as Honeycrisp or Gala)
• 1/4 cup unsweetened applesauce
• 2 tbsp chopped walnuts or pecans
• 1 tsp ground cinnamon
• 1/4 tsp ground nutmeg
• 1 tbsp maple syrup (optional)

Instructions:

1. Preheat the oven to 375°F. Lightly grease a baking dish or line it with parchment paper.

2. Core the apples, leaving a small well in the center of each one. Place the apples in the prepared baking dish.

3. In a small bowl, mix together the unsweetened applesauce, chopped nuts, cinnamon, and nutmeg.

4. Spoon the applesauce mixture into the center of each apple, dividing it evenly.

5. If desired, drizzle a small amount of maple syrup over the top of the apples.

6. Bake the apples for 25•30 minutes, or until they are tender and the filling is hot. Serve the baked apples warm, either on their own or with a dollop of plain Greek yogurt or a sprinkle of additional cinnamon.

Why this recipe is suitable for menopause:

• Apples are a good source of fiber, which can help regulate digestion during menopause.
• Cinnamon and nutmeg are warming spices that can help reduce inflammation and manage menopausal symptoms.

• Walnuts or pecans provide healthy fats and protein to support hormone balance.

• The recipe is naturally sweetened with a small amount of maple syrup, which is a better option than refined sugar.

• This dessert•like treat is low in added sugars and carbohydrates, making it a suitable option for managing blood sugar levels during menopause.

Enjoy these baked apples as a comforting and nourishing dessert or snack during the menopausal transition.

11. Shrimp and Vegetable Skewers

Ingredient:

- 2 tbsp lemon juice
- 1 tsp dried oregano
- 1/2 tsp garlic powder
- Salt and pepper to taste
- Wooden or metal skewers

- 1 lb large shrimp, peeled and deveined
- 1 red bell pepper, cut into 1•inch pieces
- 1 zucchini, cut into 1•inch pieces
- 1 red onion, cut into 1•inch pieces
- 2 tbsp olive oil

Instructions:

1. If using wooden skewers, soak them in water for 30 minutes to prevent them from burning.

2. In a large bowl, combine the shrimp, bell pepper, zucchini, and red onion.

3. In a small bowl, whisk together the olive oil, lemon juice, oregano, and garlic powder. Pour the marinade over the shrimp and vegetables and toss to coat.

4. Thread the shrimp and vegetables onto the skewers, alternating the ingredients.

5. Preheat your grill or grill pan to medium•high heat. Grill the skewers for 2•3 minutes per side, or until the shrimp are opaque and the vegetables are tender.

6. Season the grilled skewers with salt and pepper to taste. Serve the Shrimp and Vegetable Skewers hot, garnished with additional lemon wedges if desired.

Why this recipe is suitable for menopause:

- Shrimp is a lean protein source that is easy to digest and can help support muscle mass during menopause.
- The variety of vegetables, such as bell pepper, zucchini, and onion, provide a range of vitamins, minerals, and antioxidants to support overall health.
- Lemon and oregano are ingredients with anti•inflammatory properties that can help manage menopausal symptoms.
- This dish is low in carbohydrates and added sugars, making it a suitable option for maintaining stable blood sugar levels.

The Shrimp and Vegetable Skewers are a flavorful, nutrient•dense, and easy•to•prepare meal that can be enjoyed as part of a balanced menopausal diet. The grilled components and simple marinade make this a great option for a quick and healthy dinner or a summer barbecue.

12. Cauliflower Fried Rice

Ingredient:

- 1 head of cauliflower, cut into florets
- 2 tbsp sesame oil
- 1 onion, diced
- 2 cloves garlic, minced
- 1 cup frozen peas and carrots
- 2 eggs, lightly beaten
- 2 tbsp low•sodium soy sauce or tamari
- 1 tsp ground ginger
- Salt and pepper to taste
- Chopped green onions for garnish (optional)

Instructions:

1. In a food processor, pulse the cauliflower florets until they resemble the size and texture of rice grains. Set aside.

2. In a large skillet or wok, heat the sesame oil over medium•high heat. Add the diced onion and sauté for 2•3 minutes until translucent.

3. Add the minced garlic and sauté for an additional minute, until fragrant.

4. Stir in the riced cauliflower and frozen peas and carrots. Cook for 5•7 minutes, stirring occasionally, until the cauliflower is tender.

5. Push the cauliflower mixture to the side of the pan and pour the beaten eggs into the empty space. Scramble the eggs, then mix them into the cauliflower mixture.

6. Add the soy sauce or tamari and ground ginger. Stir to combine. Season the cauliflower fried rice with salt and pepper to taste. Serve the cauliflower fried rice hot, garnished with chopped green onions if desired.

Why this recipe is suitable for menopause:

- Cauliflower is a low•carb, nutrient•dense vegetable that can help support hormone balance and overall health during menopause.
- Eggs provide a source of protein to help maintain muscle mass and support bone health.
- Ginger and soy sauce are anti•inflammatory ingredients that can help manage menopausal symptoms.
- This dish is low in added sugars and carbohydrates, making it a suitable option for maintaining stable blood sugar levels.

The Cauliflower Fried Rice is a delicious, nutritious, and easy•to•prepare meal that can be enjoyed as part of a balanced menopausal diet. It's a great way to incorporate more vegetables and healthy fats into your meals during this transitional time.

13. Spinach and Feta Stuffed Chicken Breast

Ingredient:

• 4 boneless, skinless chicken breasts
• 2 cups fresh spinach, chopped
• 1/2 cup crumbled feta cheese
• 2 tbsp olive oil
• 1 tsp dried oregano
• Salt and pepper to taste

Instructions:

1. Preheat the oven to 400°F. Lightly grease a baking dish or line it with parchment paper.

2. Slice each chicken breast horizontally to create a pocket, being careful not to cut all the way through.

3. In a small bowl, mix together the chopped spinach and crumbled feta cheese.

4. Stuff the spinach and feta mixture into the pockets of the chicken breasts.

5. Drizzle the stuffed chicken breasts with olive oil and sprinkle with dried oregano, salt, and pepper.

6. Bake the stuffed chicken breasts for 25•30 minutes, or until the chicken is cooked through and the internal temperature reaches 165°F. Serve the Spinach and Feta Stuffed Chicken Breast hot, garnished with additional fresh spinach or herbs if desired.

Why this recipe is suitable for menopause:

• Chicken is a lean protein source that is easy to digest and can help support muscle mass during menopause.
• Spinach is a nutrient•dense green that is rich in vitamins, minerals, and antioxidants to support overall health.
• Feta cheese provides a source of calcium, which is important for maintaining bone health during the menopausal transition.
• Oregano is an herb with anti•inflammatory properties that can help manage menopausal symptoms.
• This dish is low in carbohydrates and added sugars, making it a suitable option for maintaining stable blood sugar levels.

The Spinach and Feta Stuffed Chicken Breast is a flavorful and nutritious meal that can be enjoyed as part of a balanced menopausal diet. The combination of protein, vegetables, and healthy fats can help support overall well•being during this transitional time.

14. Zucchini Noodles with Pesto

Ingredient:

• 3 medium zucchini, spiralized or
 julienned into noodles
• 1/2 cup basil pesto (store•bought or homemade)
• 1/4 cup toasted pine nuts
• 2 tbsp grated Parmesan cheese (optional)
• Salt and pepper to taste

For the Basil Pesto:
• 2 cups fresh basil leaves
• 1/4 cup pine nuts
• 2 cloves garlic
• 1/4 cup olive oil
• 2 tbsp grated Parmesan cheese
• Salt and pepper to taste

Instructions:

Homemade Basil Pesto:

1. In a food processor or blender, combine the basil leaves, pine nuts, and garlic. Pulse until finely chopped.
2. With the motor running, slowly drizzle in the olive oil until a smooth pesto forms.
3. Stir in the Parmesan cheese and season with salt and pepper to taste.

Zucchini Noodles with Pesto:

1. Using a spiralizer or julienne peeler, create zucchini noodles from the 3 medium zucchinis.
2. In a large bowl, toss the zucchini noodles with the basil pesto until well coated.
3. Top the zucchini noodles with the toasted pine nuts and grated Parmesan cheese (if using).
4. Season with salt and pepper to taste. Serve the Zucchini Noodles with Pesto immediately, or refrigerate until ready to serve.

Why this recipe is suitable for menopause:

• Zucchini is a low•carb, nutrient•dense vegetable that can help support hormone balance and overall health during menopause.
• Basil pesto is a source of healthy fats from the olive oil and pine nuts, which can help regulate hormone levels.
• Pine nuts and Parmesan cheese provide a boost of protein to help maintain muscle mass.
• This dish is low in added sugars and carbohydrates, making it a suitable option for managing blood sugar levels during the menopausal transition.

The Zucchini Noodles with Pesto is a refreshing, flavorful, and nutritious meal that can be enjoyed as part of a balanced menopausal diet. The versatility of this recipe also makes it a great option for a quick and easy weeknight dinner.

15. Grilled Portobello Mushrooms with Balsamic Glaze

Ingredient:

- 2 cloves garlic, minced
- 1 tsp dried thyme
- Salt and pepper to taste
- Chopped fresh parsley for garnish (optional)

- 4 large portobello mushroom caps, stems removed
- 2 tbsp olive oil
- 2 tbsp balsamic vinegar
- 1 tbsp honey

Instructions:

1. Preheat your grill or grill pan to medium•high heat.

2. In a small bowl, whisk together the olive oil, balsamic vinegar, honey, garlic, and dried thyme. Season with salt and pepper.

3. Brush the portobello mushroom caps with the balsamic glaze mixture, making sure to coat both sides.

4. Grill the mushrooms for 4•5 minutes per side, or until they are tender and slightly charred.

5. Transfer the grilled portobello mushrooms to a serving plate.

6. Drizzle any remaining balsamic glaze over the mushrooms. Garnish with chopped fresh parsley, if desired. Serve the Grilled Portobello Mushrooms with Balsamic Glaze warm.

Why this recipe is suitable for menopause:

- Portobello mushrooms are a good source of antioxidants, vitamins, and minerals that can help support overall health during menopause.

- Balsamic vinegar and honey provide a balance of acidity and natural sweetness without spiking blood sugar levels.

- Thyme is an herb with anti•inflammatory properties that can help manage menopausal symptoms.

- This dish is low in carbohydrates and high in fiber, making it a suitable option for maintaining stable blood sugar levels.

The Grilled Portobello Mushrooms with Balsamic Glaze is a simple, yet flavorful and nutritious side dish or main course that can be enjoyed as part of a balanced menopausal diet. The grilled mushrooms and tangy•sweet glaze make for a delicious and satisfying meal.

16. Tuna Salad Lettuce Wraps

Ingredient:

• 2 (5 oz) cans of tuna, drained and flaked
• 2 tbsp plain Greek yogurt
• 1 tbsp Dijon mustard
• 1 tbsp lemon juice
• 2 tbsp finely chopped celery
• 2 tbsp finely chopped red onion
• 1 tbsp chopped fresh parsley
• Salt and pepper to taste
• 8•10 large lettuce leaves (such as romaine or butter lettuce)

Instructions:

1. In a medium bowl, combine the flaked tuna, Greek yogurt, Dijon mustard, lemon juice, celery, red onion, and parsley. Mix well until fully incorporated.

2. Season the tuna salad with salt and pepper to taste.

3. Lay the lettuce leaves flat on a clean surface. Scoop a portion of the tuna salad onto the center of each lettuce leaf.

4. Fold the sides of the lettuce leaf over the tuna salad and then roll up the leaf to create a wrap. Serve the Tuna Salad Lettuce Wraps immediately, or refrigerate until ready to serve.

This recipe is suitable for menopause for the following reasons:

• Tuna is a lean protein source that can help support muscle mass and overall health during menopause.
• Greek yogurt provides a source of protein and probiotics, which can aid in digestion.
• The vegetables, such as celery and onion, offer a variety of vitamins, minerals, and antioxidants.
• Lemon juice and Dijon mustard add flavor without the need for added sugars or unhealthy fats.
• Lettuce leaves are a low•carb, nutrient•dense alternative to traditional bread or wraps, making this a suitable option for managing blood sugar levels during menopause.

The Tuna Salad Lettuce Wraps are a refreshing, flavorful, and nutritious meal or snack that can be enjoyed as part of a balanced menopausal diet. The combination of protein, vegetables, and healthy fats can help support overall well•being during this transitional time.

17. Eggplant Parmesan with Marinara Sauce

Ingredient:

- 2 cloves garlic, minced
- 1 tsp dried oregano
- Salt and pepper to taste
- Fresh basil leaves for garnish (optional)

- 2 medium eggplants, sliced into 1/2·inch thick rounds
- 2 tbsp olive oil
- 1 cup grated Parmesan cheese
- 1 cup shredded mozzarella cheese
- 1 cup marinara sauce (homemade or store·bought)

Instructions:

1. Preheat the oven to 375°F. Lightly grease a baking sheet or casserole dish.

2. Arrange the eggplant slices in a single layer on the prepared baking sheet. Brush the tops of the eggplant slices with olive oil and season with salt and pepper.

3. Bake the eggplant for 15·20 minutes, flipping halfway, until tender and lightly browned.

4. In a small bowl, mix together the Parmesan and mozzarella cheeses.

5. Spread a thin layer of marinara sauce in the bottom of the baking dish or casserole. Arrange a layer of the baked eggplant slices on top.

6. Sprinkle the eggplant layer with some of the garlic, oregano, and the cheese mixture.

7. Repeat the layers of eggplant, sauce, garlic, oregano, and cheese until all the ingredients are used up, ending with the cheese mixture.

8. Bake the Eggplant Parmesan for 20·25 minutes, or until the cheese is melted and bubbly. Remove from the oven and let cool for 5 minutes before serving. Garnish with fresh basil leaves, if desired.

Why this recipe is suitable for menopause:

- Eggplant is a low·carb, fiber·rich vegetable that can help support digestive health during menopause.
- Parmesan and mozzarella cheeses provide a source of calcium, which is important for maintaining bone health.
- Garlic and oregano are anti·inflammatory ingredients that can help manage menopausal symptoms.

The Eggplant Parmesan with Marinara Sauce is a comforting, nutrient·dense meal that can be enjoyed as part of a balanced menopausal diet. The combination of vegetables, cheese, and herbs creates a flavorful and satisfying dish.

18. Broccoli and Cheese Stuffed Peppers

Ingredient:

• 4 medium bell peppers, halved lengthwise and seeds removed
• 1 cup chopped broccoli florets
• 1/2 cup shredded cheddar cheese
• 1/4 cup grated Parmesan cheese
• 2 tbsp plain Greek yogurt
• 1 clove garlic, minced
• 1 tsp dried oregano
• Salt and pepper to taste

Instructions:

1. Preheat your oven to 375°F. Lightly grease a baking dish or line it with parchment paper.

2. Arrange the bell pepper halves in the prepared baking dish, cut•side up.

3. In a medium bowl, combine the chopped broccoli, cheddar cheese, Parmesan cheese, Greek yogurt, garlic, and oregano. Mix well.

4. Spoon the broccoli and cheese mixture evenly into the bell pepper halves.

5. Bake the stuffed peppers for 25•30 minutes, or until the peppers are tender and the filling is hot and bubbly.

6. Remove the Broccoli and Cheese Stuffed Peppers from the oven and let cool for 5 minutes before serving. Season with salt and pepper to taste.

Why this recipe is suitable for menopause:

• Bell peppers are a good source of vitamins C and A, which can help support immune function and skin health during menopause.
• Broccoli is a nutrient•dense vegetable that provides fiber, antioxidants, and anti•inflammatory compounds to help manage menopausal symptoms.
• Cheddar and Parmesan cheeses are a source of calcium, which is important for maintaining bone health.
• Greek yogurt adds protein and probiotics to support digestive health.
• This dish is relatively low in carbohydrates and high in fiber, making it a suitable option for managing blood sugar levels during the menopausal transition.

19. Avocado Tuna Salad

Ingredient:

• 2 (5 oz) cans of tuna, drained
• 1 ripe avocado, diced
• 2 tbsp plain Greek yogurt
• 1 tbsp lemon juice
• 2 tbsp finely chopped celery
• 2 tbsp finely chopped red onion
• 1 tbsp chopped fresh parsley
• Salt and pepper to taste

Instructions:

1. In a medium bowl, gently mix together the drained tuna, diced avocado, Greek yogurt, and lemon juice until well combined.

2. Fold in the chopped celery, red onion, and parsley.

3. Season the avocado tuna salad with salt and pepper to taste.

4. Serve the avocado tuna salad on its own, on top of mixed greens, or with whole grain crackers or slices of cucumber.

This recipe is suitable for menopause for the following reasons:

• Tuna is a lean protein source that can help support muscle mass and overall health during menopause.
• Avocado is a good source of healthy monounsaturated fats, which can help regulate hormone levels and reduce inflammation.
• Greek yogurt provides a source of protein and probiotics to support digestive health.
• The vegetables, such as celery and onion, offer a variety of vitamins, minerals, and antioxidants.
• This salad is low in carbohydrates and added sugars, making it a suitable option for maintaining stable blood sugar levels during the menopausal transition.

The Avocado Tuna Salad is a nutrient•dense, flavorful, and versatile dish that can be enjoyed as a light meal, snack, or topping. The combination of protein, healthy fats, and antioxidants makes it a great choice to support overall health and well•being during menopause.

20. Baked Cod with Herbs

Ingredient:

- 4 (6 oz) cod fillets
- 2 tbsp olive oil
- 2 tbsp chopped fresh parsley
- 1 tbsp chopped fresh dill
- 1 tbsp chopped fresh thyme
- 2 cloves garlic, minced
- 1 tsp lemon zest
- Salt and pepper to taste

Instructions:

1. Preheat your oven to 400°F. Lightly grease a baking dish or line it with parchment paper.

2. Place the cod fillets in the prepared baking dish.

3. In a small bowl, mix together the olive oil, parsley, dill, thyme, garlic, and lemon zest.

4. Spoon the herb mixture over the top of the cod fillets, making sure to evenly distribute it.

5. Season the cod with salt and pepper to taste.

6. Bake the cod for 15•20 minutes, or until it flakes easily with a fork and is opaque throughout. Serve the Baked Cod with Herbs immediately, garnished with additional fresh herbs if desired.

The Baked Cod with Herbs is a simple, yet flavorful and nutritious meal that can be enjoyed as part of a balanced menopausal diet. The baked preparation and herb•infused topping make this an easy and versatile option for a quick weeknight dinner or a more formal meal.

21. Quinoa and Black Bean Salad

Ingredient:

• 1 cup uncooked quinoa, rinsed
• 1 (15 oz) can black beans, rinsed and drained
• 1 cup diced cucumber
• 1 cup diced tomatoes
• 1/2 cup diced red onion
• 1/4 cup chopped fresh cilantro
• 2 tbsp olive oil
• 2 tbsp lime juice
• 1 tsp ground cumin
• 1/2 tsp chili powder
• Salt and pepper to taste

Instructions:
1. Cook the quinoa according to package instructions. Allow to cool completely.

2. In a large bowl, combine the cooked quinoa, black beans, cucumber, tomatoes, red onion, and cilantro.

3. In a small bowl, whisk together the olive oil, lime juice, cumin, and chili powder.

4. Pour the dressing over the quinoa and bean mixture and toss gently to coat.

5. Season the salad with salt and pepper to taste.

6. Refrigerate the Quinoa and Black Bean Salad for at least 30 minutes to allow the flavors to meld. Serve chilled or at room temperature.

This salad is suitable for menopause for the following reasons:

• Quinoa is a gluten•free, high•protein grain that can help support muscle mass and energy levels during menopause.
• Black beans are a good source of fiber, protein, and complex carbohydrates, which can help regulate blood sugar levels.
• The vegetables, such as cucumber, tomatoes, and onion, provide a variety of vitamins, minerals, and antioxidants to support overall health.
• Cilantro, lime juice, cumin, and chili powder add flavor and anti•inflammatory properties to the dish.

22. Chicken and Vegetable Kebabs

Ingredient:

- 1 lb boneless, skinless chicken breasts, cut into 1·inch cubes
- 1 red bell pepper, cut into 1·inch pieces
- 1 zucchini, cut into 1·inch pieces
- 1 red onion, cut into 1·inch pieces
- 8 oz cremini or button mushrooms, halved
- 2 tbsp olive oil
- 2 tbsp lemon juice
- 1 tsp dried oregano
- 1/2 tsp garlic powder
- Salt and pepper to taste
- Wooden or metal skewers

Instructions:

1. If using wooden skewers, soak them in water for 30 minutes to prevent them from burning.

2. In a large bowl, combine the cubed chicken, bell pepper, zucchini, red onion, and mushrooms.

3. In a small bowl, whisk together the olive oil, lemon juice, oregano, and garlic powder. Pour the marinade over the chicken and vegetables and toss to coat.

4. Thread the marinated chicken and vegetables onto the skewers, alternating the ingredients.

5. Preheat your grill or grill pan to medium·high heat.

6. Grill the chicken and vegetable kebabs for 12·15 minutes, turning occasionally, until the chicken is cooked through and the vegetables are tender.

7. Season the grilled kebabs with salt and pepper to taste. Serve the Chicken and Vegetable Kebabs hot, with any remaining marinade drizzled over the top.

The Chicken and Vegetable Kebabs are a flavorful, nutrient·dense, and easy·to·prepare meal that can be enjoyed as part of a balanced menopausal diet. The grilled components and simple marinade make this a great option for a quick and healthy dinner or a summer barbecue.

23. Stir•Fried Tofu with Vegetables

Ingredient:

• 1 block (14 oz) extra•firm tofu, pressed and cubed
• 2 tbsp sesame oil
• 1 red bell pepper, sliced
• 1 cup broccoli florets
• 1 cup sliced mushrooms
• 1 cup snow peas or snap peas
• 2 cloves garlic, minced
• 1 tbsp grated fresh ginger
• 2 tbsp low•sodium soy sauce or tamari
• 1 tsp sesame seeds (optional)
• Salt and pepper to taste

Instructions:

1. In a large skillet or wok, heat the sesame oil over medium•high heat.

2. Add the cubed tofu and stir•fry for 3•4 minutes, until lightly browned on all sides. Transfer the tofu to a plate and set aside.

3. In the same skillet, add the sliced bell pepper, broccoli, mushrooms, and snow peas. Stir•fry for 4•5 minutes, until the vegetables are tender•crisp.

4. Add the minced garlic and grated ginger to the skillet. Cook for 1 minute, until fragrant.

5. Return the sautéed tofu to the skillet. Pour in the soy sauce or tamari and toss everything together until well combined.

6. Remove the stir•fried tofu and vegetables from the heat. Sprinkle with sesame seeds, if desired.

7. Season the dish with salt and pepper to taste. Serve the Stir•Fried Tofu with Vegetables hot, over steamed brown rice or quinoa, if desired.

Why this recipe is suitable for menopause:

• Tofu is a plant•based protein source that is gentle on the digestive system and can help support muscle mass during menopause.
• The variety of vegetables, such as bell pepper, broccoli, mushrooms, and snow peas, provide a range of vitamins, minerals, and antioxidants to support overall health.

24. Mediterranean Chickpea Salad

Ingredient:

• 2 (15 oz) cans chickpeas, drained and rinsed
• 1 cup cherry tomatoes, halved
• 1/2 cup diced cucumber
• 1/4 cup diced red onion
• 1/4 cup crumbled feta cheese
• 2 tbsp chopped fresh parsley
• 2 tbsp olive oil
• 2 tbsp red wine vinegar
• 1 tsp dried oregano
• 1/4 tsp salt
• 1/4 tsp black pepper

Instructions:

1. In a large bowl, combine the drained and rinsed chickpeas, halved cherry tomatoes, diced cucumber, diced red onion, crumbled feta cheese, and chopped fresh parsley.

2. In a small bowl, whisk together the olive oil, red wine vinegar, dried oregano, salt, and black pepper.

3. Pour the dressing over the chickpea salad and toss gently to coat.

4. Cover and refrigerate for at least 30 minutes to allow the flavors to meld.

5. Serve chilled or at room temperature.

This Mediterranean Chickpea Salad is a great option for the Galveston Diet and menopausal women. Chickpeas are a good source of plant•based protein, fiber, and complex carbohydrates, which can help manage blood sugar levels. The healthy fats from the olive oil and the antioxidants from the vegetables make this a nutritious and satisfying dish.

The combination of flavors, including the tangy vinegar, aromatic oregano, and salty feta, creates a delicious and balanced salad that can be enjoyed as a main course or a side dish. It's also easy to prepare and can be made in advance, making it a convenient option for busy menopausal women.

25. Baked Garlic Herb Chicken Thighs

Ingredient:

- 8 bone•in, skin•on chicken thighs
- 3 tbsp olive oil
- 4 cloves garlic, minced
- 2 tsp dried oregano
- 1 tsp dried thyme
- 1 tsp paprika
- 1/2 tsp salt
- 1/4 tsp black pepper

Instructions:

1. Preheat your oven to 400°F. Line a baking sheet with parchment paper or foil.

2. In a small bowl, mix together the olive oil, minced garlic, oregano, thyme, paprika, salt, and pepper.

3. Place the chicken thighs skin•side up on the prepared baking sheet. Brush or rub the garlic•herb mixture all over the chicken, making sure to coat the skin well.

4. Bake the chicken for 35•40 minutes, or until the internal temperature reaches 165°F. The skin should be crispy and golden brown.

5. Remove the chicken from the oven and let it rest for 5 minutes before serving.

This recipe is perfect for the Galveston Diet as it is high in protein, low in carbs, and uses healthy fats from the olive oil. The garlic, herbs, and spices provide a flavorful boost without adding any unnecessary sugars or processed ingredients.

The chicken thighs are a great choice for menopausal women as they are a good source of iron, which can help combat fatigue and anemia. The dish is also easy to prepare and can be enjoyed as a main course or added to salads or vegetable dishes.

26. Ratatouille

Ingredient:

• 1 medium eggplant, diced
• 1 medium zucchini, diced
• 1 medium yellow squash, diced
• 1 red bell pepper, diced
• 1 onion, diced
• 3 cloves garlic, minced
• 2 tbsp olive oil
• 1 (14.5 oz) can diced tomatoes
• 2 tbsp chopped fresh basil
• 1 tsp dried oregano
• Salt and pepper to taste

Instructions:

1. In a large skillet or Dutch oven, heat the olive oil over medium heat.

2. Add the diced eggplant, zucchini, yellow squash, bell pepper, and onion. Sauté for 8•10 minutes, stirring occasionally, until the vegetables are tender.

3. Stir in the minced garlic and cook for an additional 1•2 minutes, until fragrant.

4. Pour in the can of diced tomatoes, including the juices. Add the chopped basil and dried oregano.

5. Bring the ratatouille to a simmer and let it cook for 15•20 minutes, stirring occasionally, until the flavors have melded and the sauce has thickened slightly.

6. Season the ratatouille with salt and pepper to taste. Serve the Ratatouille warm, garnished with additional fresh basil if desired.

Why this recipe is suitable for menopause:

• Eggplant, zucchini, and bell pepper are low•carb, fiber•rich vegetables that can help support digestive health during menopause.
• Tomatoes are a good source of lycopene, an antioxidant that may help reduce the risk of certain health issues associated with menopause.
• Basil and oregano are herbs with anti•inflammatory properties that can help manage menopausal symptoms.

27. Cucumber and Tomato Salad with Feta

Ingredient:

• 2 large cucumbers, peeled, seeded and diced
• 2 cups cherry or grape tomatoes, halved
• 1/2 red onion, thinly sliced
• 1/2 cup crumbled feta cheese
• 2 tbsp olive oil
• 2 tbsp red wine vinegar
• 1 tbsp lemon juice
• 1 tsp dried oregano
• 1/4 tsp salt
• 1/4 tsp black pepper

Instructions:

1. In a large bowl, combine the diced cucumbers, halved tomatoes, and sliced red onion.

2. In a small bowl, whisk together the olive oil, red wine vinegar, lemon juice, oregano, salt and pepper.

3. Pour the dressing over the cucumber and tomato mixture and toss gently to coat.

4. Sprinkle the crumbled feta cheese over the top.

5. Refrigerate for at least 30 minutes to allow the flavors to meld.

6. Serve chilled or at room temperature.

This salad is perfect for the Galveston Diet as it is packed with hydrating vegetables, healthy fats from the olive oil and feta, and is low in carbs. The combination of cucumbers, tomatoes, and feta provides a refreshing and flavorful dish that is suitable for managing menopausal symptoms. Enjoy!

28. Stuffed Acorn Squash with Quinoa and Cranberries

Ingredient:

• 2 acorn squash, halved and seeded
• 1 cup quinoa, rinsed
• 2 cups vegetable or chicken broth
• 1/2 cup dried cranberries
• 1/4 cup chopped pecans
• 2 tbsp maple syrup
• 1 tsp ground cinnamon
• 1/4 tsp ground nutmeg
• Salt and pepper to taste

Instructions:

1. Preheat oven to 400°F. Place the acorn squash halves cut•side up on a baking sheet. Bake for 30•40 minutes, until tender when pierced with a fork.

2. Meanwhile, in a medium saucepan, combine the quinoa and broth. Bring to a boil, then reduce heat to low, cover and simmer for 15•20 minutes, until quinoa is cooked through. Fluff with a fork.

3. In a medium bowl, mix the cooked quinoa, cranberries, pecans, maple syrup, cinnamon, nutmeg, salt and pepper.

4. Scoop the quinoa mixture evenly into the baked acorn squash halves.

5. Return the stuffed squash to the oven and bake for an additional 10•15 minutes, until heated through.

6. Serve the stuffed acorn squash warm. Enjoy!

The sweet and savory flavors of the quinoa, cranberries, and spices pair perfectly with the roasted acorn squash. This makes a great vegetarian main dish or side.

29. Lemon Garlic Shrimp with Asparagus

Ingredient:

• 1 lb large shrimp, peeled and deveined
• 1 lb asparagus, trimmed and cut into 1·inch pieces
• 3 tbsp olive oil
• 4 cloves garlic, minced
• 2 tbsp lemon juice
• 1 tsp lemon zest
• 1/4 tsp red pepper flakes (optional)
• Salt and black pepper to taste
• 2 tbsp chopped fresh parsley

Instructions:

1. In a large skillet, heat the olive oil over medium·high heat. Add the minced garlic and cook for 1 minute, until fragrant.

2. Add the shrimp and asparagus to the skillet. Season with salt and black pepper. Cook, stirring occasionally, for 5·7 minutes, until the shrimp are opaque and the asparagus is tender·crisp.

3. Remove the skillet from the heat and stir in the lemon juice, lemon zest, and red pepper flakes (if using).

4. Sprinkle the chopped fresh parsley over the top.

5. Serve immediately, while hot.

This Lemon Garlic Shrimp with Asparagus dish is an excellent choice for the Galveston Diet and menopausal women. Shrimp is a lean protein that is low in calories and high in nutrients, while asparagus is a nutrient·dense vegetable that is rich in fiber, vitamins, and antioxidants.

The lemon and garlic flavors provide a bright, zesty taste that complements the shrimp and asparagus perfectly. The dish is also low in carbs and high in healthy fats from the olive oil, making it a great option for managing blood sugar levels and supporting overall health during menopause.

This recipe is easy to prepare and can be served as a main dish or a side. It's a versatile and nutritious option that can be enjoyed by the whole family.

30. Berry and Spinach Salad with Goat Cheese

Ingredient:

- 5 oz baby spinach
- 1 cup mixed berries (such as blueberries, raspberries, and strawberries)
- 2 oz crumbled goat cheese
- 2 tbsp chopped walnuts
- 1 tbsp balsamic vinegar
- 1 tbsp olive oil
- 1 tsp Dijon mustard
- 1 tsp honey
- Salt and pepper to taste

Instructions:

1. In a large salad bowl, combine the baby spinach, mixed berries, crumbled goat cheese, and chopped walnuts.

2. In a small bowl, whisk together the balsamic vinegar, olive oil, Dijon mustard, and honey until well combined.

3. Drizzle the balsamic vinaigrette over the salad and toss gently to coat. Season the Berry and Spinach Salad with Goat Cheese with salt and pepper to taste. Serve the salad immediately, or refrigerate until ready to serve.

Why this recipe is suitable for menopause:

- Spinach is a nutrient•dense green that is rich in vitamins, minerals, and antioxidants to support overall health during menopause.
- Berries are a good source of fiber, vitamins, and antioxidants that can help reduce inflammation and manage menopausal symptoms.
- Goat cheese provides a source of calcium, which is important for maintaining bone health.
- Walnuts are a healthy source of omega•3 fatty acids that can help regulate hormone levels.
- The balsamic vinaigrette is low in added sugars and provides a balance of acidity and sweetness without spiking blood sugar levels.

The Berry and Spinach Salad with Goat Cheese is a refreshing, flavorful, and nutrient•dense meal that can be enjoyed as part of a balanced menopausal diet. The combination of greens, berries, cheese, and nuts makes it a satisfying and well•rounded option.

31. Greek Chicken Souvlaki with Tzatziki Sauce

Ingredient:

Chicken Souvlaki:
• 1 lb boneless, skinless chicken breasts, cut into 1•inch cubes
• 2 tbsp olive oil
• 2 tbsp lemon juice
• 2 garlic cloves, minced
• 1 tsp dried oregano
• 1/2 tsp salt
• 1/4 tsp black pepper

Tzatziki Sauce:
• 1 cup plain Greek yogurt
• 1 cucumber, peeled, seeded and grated
• 2 garlic cloves, minced
• 1 tbsp lemon juice
• 1 tbsp chopped fresh dill
• 1/4 tsp salt

Instructions:

1. Make the Chicken Souvlaki:
• In a large bowl, combine the chicken, olive oil, lemon juice, garlic, oregano, salt and pepper. Toss to coat the chicken evenly. Cover and marinate in the refrigerator for 30 minutes to 1 hour.

2. Make the Tzatziki Sauce:
• In a medium bowl, mix together the yogurt, grated cucumber, garlic, lemon juice, dill and salt. Cover and refrigerate until ready to serve.

3. Assemble the Souvlaki:
• Thread the marinated chicken cubes onto skewers.
• Grill the skewers over medium•high heat for 8•10 minutes, turning occasionally, until the chicken is cooked through.

4. Serve:
• Serve the grilled chicken souvlaki with the tzatziki sauce on the side. Enjoy with pita bread, rice or a fresh Greek salad.

32. Butternut Squash Soup

Ingredient:

• 1 medium butternut squash, peeled, seeded, and cubed (about 4 cups)
• 1 onion, diced
• 2 cloves garlic, minced
• 4 cups low•sodium vegetable or chicken broth
• 1 tsp ground cumin
• 1/2 tsp ground cinnamon
• 1/4 tsp ground nutmeg
• Salt and pepper to taste
• 2 tbsp plain Greek yogurt (optional)
• Chopped fresh parsley for garnish (optional)

Instructions:

1. In a large pot or Dutch oven, sauté the diced onion in a small amount of olive oil over medium heat until translucent, about 5 minutes.

2. Add the minced garlic and sauté for an additional 1 minute, until fragrant.

3. Add the cubed butternut squash and broth to the pot. Bring the mixture to a boil.

4. Reduce the heat to low, cover, and simmer for 20•25 minutes, or until the squash is very soft.

5. Remove the pot from the heat and use an immersion blender to puree the soup until smooth. Alternatively, you can transfer the soup to a blender in batches and blend until creamy.

6. Stir in the ground cumin, cinnamon, and nutmeg. Season the soup with salt and pepper to taste.

7. Serve the Butternut Squash Soup warm, garnished with a dollop of plain Greek yogurt and chopped fresh parsley, if desired.

The Butternut Squash Soup is a comforting, nourishing, and easy•to•prepare meal that can be enjoyed as part of a balanced menopausal diet. The creamy texture and warm spices make it a delicious and satisfying option.

33. Beet and Goat Cheese Salad

Ingredient:

• 4 medium beets, peeled and sliced into wedges
• 2 tbsp olive oil
• 1 tbsp balsamic vinegar
• 1 tsp Dijon mustard
• 1 tsp honey
• Salt and pepper to taste
• 5 oz mixed greens
• 1/2 cup crumbled goat cheese
• 2 tbsp chopped walnuts

Instructions:

1. Preheat your oven to 400°F. Toss the beet wedges with 1 tbsp of the olive oil and season with salt and pepper. Spread the beets on a baking sheet and roast for 20•25 minutes, until tender.

2. In a small bowl, whisk together the remaining 1 tbsp olive oil, balsamic vinegar, Dijon mustard, and honey. Season with salt and pepper to taste.

3. In a large salad bowl, combine the roasted beet wedges, mixed greens, crumbled goat cheese, and chopped walnuts.

4. Drizzle the balsamic vinaigrette over the salad and toss gently to coat.

5. Serve the Beet and Goat Cheese Salad immediately.

This salad is an excellent choice for the Galveston Diet and menopausal women. Beets are a nutrient•dense vegetable that are rich in antioxidants, fiber, and folate, which can help support overall health during menopause. The goat cheese provides a creamy, tangy contrast to the sweet beets, while the walnuts add a satisfying crunch.

The balsamic vinaigrette dressing is made with healthy fats from the olive oil and a touch of honey for sweetness, without any added sugars. This combination of ingredients makes for a balanced and flavorful salad that is suitable for managing menopausal symptoms and supporting a healthy lifestyle.

This salad can be enjoyed as a main dish or a side, and it's easy to prepare in advance, making it a convenient option for busy menopausal women.

34. Sautéed Brussels Sprouts with Bacon

Ingredient:

• 1 lb Brussels sprouts, trimmed and halved
• 4 slices bacon, chopped
• 2 tbsp olive oil
• 2 cloves garlic, minced
• 1/4 tsp red pepper flakes (optional)
• Salt and pepper to taste

Instructions:

1. In a large skillet, cook the chopped bacon over medium heat until crispy, about 5•7 minutes. Transfer the cooked bacon to a paper towel•lined plate, reserving the bacon fat in the skillet.

2. Add the olive oil to the skillet with the reserved bacon fat. Increase the heat to medium•high and add the halved Brussels sprouts. Sauté for 5•7 minutes, stirring occasionally, until the Brussels sprouts are starting to brown and become tender.

3. Add the minced garlic and red pepper flakes (if using) to the skillet. Cook for an additional 1•2 minutes, until the garlic is fragrant.

4. Remove the skillet from the heat and stir in the cooked bacon. Season with salt and pepper to taste.

5. Serve the Sautéed Brussels Sprouts with Bacon warm.

This dish is an excellent choice for the Galveston Diet and menopausal women. Brussels sprouts are a nutrient•dense vegetable that are high in fiber, vitamins, and antioxidants, which can help support overall health during menopause. The addition of bacon provides a savory, satisfying flavor, while the olive oil and garlic add healthy fats and aromatic notes.

The Sautéed Brussels Sprouts with Bacon is low in carbs and high in healthy fats and protein, making it a great option for managing blood sugar levels and supporting a balanced diet. The red pepper flakes can also provide a slight kick of heat, which may help alleviate some menopausal symptoms.

This dish is easy to prepare and can be enjoyed as a side or a main course. It's a versatile and nutritious option that can be enjoyed by the whole family.

35. Baked Halibut with Mango Salsa

Ingredient:

Mango Salsa:
• 1 ripe mango, diced
• 1/2 red onion, finely chopped
• 1 jalapeño, seeded and finely chopped
• 1 tbsp fresh cilantro, chopped
• 1 tbsp lime juice
• 1/4 tsp salt

Halibut:
• 4 (6 oz) halibut fillets
• 2 tbsp olive oil
• 1 tsp garlic powder
• 1 tsp paprika
• 1/2 tsp salt
• 1/4 tsp black pepper

Instructions:

1. Preheat your oven to 400°F. Line a baking sheet with parchment paper or foil.

2. Make the mango salsa: In a medium bowl, combine the diced mango, chopped red onion, jalapeño, cilantro, lime juice, and salt. Stir to mix well and set aside.

3. Pat the halibut fillets dry with paper towels and place them on the prepared baking sheet. Drizzle the olive oil over the top and sprinkle with the garlic powder, paprika, salt, and black pepper.

4. Bake the halibut for 12•15 minutes, or until it flakes easily with a fork and reaches an internal temperature of 145°F.

5. Serve the baked halibut immediately, topped with the fresh mango salsa.

This Baked Halibut with Mango Salsa is an excellent choice for the Galveston Diet and menopausal women. Halibut is a lean, high•protein fish that is rich in omega•3 fatty acids, which can help support heart health and reduce inflammation.

The mango salsa provides a sweet and tangy contrast to the savory halibut, while also adding a boost of vitamins, minerals, and antioxidants. The combination of the baked halibut and the fresh salsa makes for a light, flavorful, and nutritious meal.

This dish is low in carbs and high in healthy fats, making it a great option for managing blood sugar levels and supporting overall health during menopause. It's also easy to prepare and can be enjoyed as a main course or a side dish.

36. Caprese Salad with Balsamic Glaze

Ingredient:

• 8 oz fresh mozzarella cheese, sliced
• 2 large tomatoes, sliced
• 1/4 cup fresh basil leaves
• 2 tbsp balsamic vinegar
• 1 tbsp honey
• 1 tbsp olive oil
• 1/4 tsp salt
• 1/8 tsp black pepper

Instructions:

1. Arrange the sliced mozzarella and tomatoes on a serving platter or plate. Scatter the fresh basil leaves over the top.

2. In a small saucepan, combine the balsamic vinegar and honey. Bring to a simmer over medium heat, stirring occasionally, until the mixture has reduced by about half and thickened slightly, about 5•7 minutes. Remove from heat and let cool slightly.

3. Drizzle the balsamic glaze over the Caprese salad.

4. Drizzle the olive oil over the top and season with salt and black pepper.

5. Serve the Caprese salad immediately, or refrigerate until ready to serve.

This Caprese Salad with Balsamic Glaze is a classic and refreshing dish that is perfect for warm weather. The combination of juicy tomatoes, creamy mozzarella, and fragrant basil is elevated by the sweet and tangy balsamic glaze.

This salad is a great option for the Galveston Diet and menopausal women as it is low in carbs, high in healthy fats from the olive oil and mozzarella, and provides a good source of antioxidants from the tomatoes and basil.

The balsamic glaze adds a touch of sweetness without any added sugars, making it a more nutritious alternative to traditional balsamic vinaigrette. This salad can be enjoyed as a light main course or a side dish, and it's easy to prepare in advance.

37. Chicken Zoodle Soup

Ingredient:

• 1 lb boneless, skinless chicken breasts, cut into 1·inch pieces
• 4 cups low·sodium chicken broth
• 2 cups water
• 2 medium zucchini, spiralized or julienned into noodles
• 1 cup sliced mushrooms
• 1/2 cup diced onion
• 2 cloves garlic, minced
• 1 tsp dried thyme
• 1/2 tsp dried oregano
• Salt and pepper to taste
• 2 tbsp chopped fresh parsley (for garnish)

Instructions:

1. In a large pot or Dutch oven, combine the chicken broth and water. Bring to a boil over high heat.

2. Add the diced chicken, sliced mushrooms, diced onion, and minced garlic to the pot. Reduce heat to medium·low and simmer for 10·12 minutes, until the chicken is cooked through.

3. Stir in the spiralized or julienned zucchini noodles, dried thyme, and dried oregano. Season with salt and pepper to taste.

4. Simmer the soup for an additional 5·7 minutes, until the zucchini noodles are tender but still have a bit of bite. Ladle the Chicken Zoodle Soup into bowls and garnish with chopped fresh parsley.

This Chicken Zoodle Soup is an excellent choice for the Galveston Diet and menopausal women. It's a low·carb, high·protein dish that is packed with nutrient·dense vegetables and lean chicken.

The zucchini noodles provide a satisfying, pasta·like texture without the added carbs, while the chicken and broth offer a comforting, nourishing base. The herbs and spices add flavor without the need for excessive sodium or sugar.

This soup is easy to prepare and can be made in advance, making it a convenient and healthy option for busy menopausal women. It's also a great way to incorporate more vegetables into your diet and support overall health during menopause.

38. Spicy Roasted Cauliflower

Ingredient:

- 1 head of cauliflower, cut into florets
- 2 tbsp olive oil
- 1 tsp paprika
- 1 tsp chili powder
- 1/2 tsp garlic powder
- 1/4 tsp cayenne pepper (or to taste)
- 1/4 tsp salt
- 1/4 tsp black pepper

Instructions:

1. Preheat your oven to 400°F. Line a baking sheet with parchment paper or a silicone baking mat.

2. In a large bowl, toss the cauliflower florets with the olive oil, paprika, chili powder, garlic powder, cayenne pepper, salt, and black pepper until the cauliflower is evenly coated.

3. Spread the seasoned cauliflower florets in a single layer on the prepared baking sheet.

4. Roast the cauliflower for 20•25 minutes, flipping halfway through, until the florets are tender and lightly browned.

5. Serve the Spicy Roasted Cauliflower warm, as a side dish or snack.

This Spicy Roasted Cauliflower is an excellent choice for the Galveston Diet and menopausal women. Cauliflower is a low•carb, nutrient•dense vegetable that is rich in fiber, vitamins, and antioxidants, which can help support overall health during menopause.

The combination of spices, including paprika, chili powder, and cayenne pepper, adds a flavorful kick to the roasted cauliflower without the need for excessive sodium or sugar. The healthy fats from the olive oil also help to make this dish more satisfying and satiating.

This recipe is easy to prepare and can be enjoyed as a side dish or a snack. It's a versatile and nutritious option that can be customized to your personal spice preference. The Spicy Roasted Cauliflower is also a great way to incorporate more vegetables into your diet during menopause.

39. Quinoa and Kale Stuffed Sweet Potatoes

Ingredient:

• 4 medium sweet potatoes, scrubbed clean
• 1 cup cooked quinoa
• 1 cup chopped kale, stems removed
• 1/4 cup crumbled feta cheese
• 2 tbsp olive oil
• 1 clove garlic, minced
• 1/4 tsp ground cumin
• 1/4 tsp paprika
• Salt and pepper to taste

Instructions:

1. Preheat your oven to 400°F. Pierce the sweet potatoes several times with a fork and place them directly on the oven rack. Bake for 45•60 minutes, until tender when pierced with a fork.

2. Remove the sweet potatoes from the oven and let them cool slightly. Cut each potato in half lengthwise.

3. In a medium bowl, combine the cooked quinoa, chopped kale, crumbled feta, olive oil, minced garlic, cumin, paprika, salt, and pepper. Mix well.

4. Scoop the quinoa and kale mixture evenly into the baked sweet potato halves.

5. Return the stuffed sweet potatoes to the oven and bake for an additional 10•15 minutes, until the filling is heated through. Serve the Quinoa and Kale Stuffed Sweet Potatoes warm.

This dish is an excellent choice for the Galveston Diet and menopausal women. Sweet potatoes are a nutrient•dense carbohydrate that are high in fiber, vitamins, and antioxidants, which can help support overall health during menopause.

The quinoa and kale provide a protein•rich, fiber•filled filling that is low in carbs and high in nutrients. The feta cheese adds a creamy, tangy flavor that complements the sweet potatoes and the other ingredients.

This recipe is easy to prepare and can be enjoyed as a main dish or a side. It's a versatile and nutritious option that can be customized to your personal taste preferences. The Quinoa and Kale Stuffed Sweet Potatoes are a great way to incorporate more plant•based, nutrient•dense foods into your diet during menopause.

40. Mediterranean Stuffed Peppers

Ingredient:

• 4 bell peppers (any color), halved lengthwise and seeds removed
• 1 cup cooked quinoa
• 1 (15 oz) can diced tomatoes, drained
• 1/2 cup crumbled feta cheese
• 1/4 cup chopped kalamata olives
• 2 tbsp chopped fresh parsley
• 1 tbsp olive oil
• 2 cloves garlic, minced
• 1 tsp dried oregano
• 1/4 tsp salt
• 1/4 tsp black pepper

Instructions:

1. Preheat your oven to 375°F. Place the bell pepper halves cut•side up in a baking dish.

2. In a medium bowl, combine the cooked quinoa, drained diced tomatoes, crumbled feta, chopped olives, parsley, olive oil, minced garlic, dried oregano, salt, and black pepper. Mix well.

3. Spoon the quinoa mixture evenly into the bell pepper halves, packing it down gently.

4. Cover the baking dish with foil and bake for 30•35 minutes, until the peppers are tender. Remove the foil and bake for an additional 5•10 minutes, until the tops are lightly browned. Serve the Mediterranean Stuffed Peppers warm.

These Mediterranean Stuffed Peppers are an excellent choice for the Galveston Diet and menopausal women. Bell peppers are a nutrient•dense vegetable that are high in vitamins, minerals, and antioxidants, which can help support overall health during menopause.

The quinoa, feta, and olives provide a flavorful, protein•rich filling that is low in carbs and high in healthy fats. The combination of Mediterranean•inspired ingredients, such as tomatoes, garlic, and oregano, adds a delicious and satisfying flavor profile to the dish.

This recipe is easy to prepare and can be made in advance, making it a convenient and nutritious option for busy menopausal women. The stuffed peppers can be enjoyed as a main course or a side dish, and they are a great way to incorporate more plant•based, nutrient•dense foods into your diet.

41. Pesto Zucchini Noodles with Cherry Tomatoes

Ingredient:

• 3 medium zucchini, spiralized or julienned into noodles
• 1 cup cherry tomatoes, halved
• 1/4 cup basil pesto (store•bought or homemade)
• 2 tbsp pine nuts (or chopped walnuts)
• 2 tbsp grated Parmesan cheese
• 1 tbsp olive oil
• Salt and pepper to taste

Instructions:

1. In a large bowl, combine the spiralized or julienned zucchini noodles and halved cherry tomatoes.

2. In a small bowl, mix together the basil pesto, pine nuts (or walnuts), and Parmesan cheese.

3. Drizzle the olive oil over the zucchini noodles and tomatoes, then toss to coat.

4. Add the pesto mixture to the zucchini noodle mixture and toss gently to combine.

5. Season with salt and pepper to taste.

6. Serve the Pesto Zucchini Noodles with Cherry Tomatoes immediately, or refrigerate until ready to serve.

This Pesto Zucchini Noodles with Cherry Tomatoes dish is an excellent choice for the Galveston Diet and menopausal women. Zucchini noodles are a low•carb, nutrient•dense alternative to traditional pasta, providing a good source of fiber, vitamins, and minerals.

The basil pesto adds a flavorful, nutrient•rich sauce that is high in healthy fats from the olive oil and pine nuts (or walnuts). The cherry tomatoes provide a burst of sweetness and antioxidants, while the Parmesan cheese adds a creamy, savory element.

This recipe is easy to prepare and can be enjoyed as a main dish or a side. It's a versatile and nutritious option that can be customized to your personal taste preferences. The Pesto Zucchini Noodles with Cherry Tomatoes are a great way to incorporate more plant•based, low•carb foods into your diet during menopause.

42. Salmon Cakes with Avocado Sauce

Ingredient:

Salmon Cakes:
• 1 (15 oz) can wild•caught salmon, drained and flaked
• 1 egg, beaten
• 1/4 cup almond flour
• 2 tbsp chopped fresh parsley
• 1 tbsp lemon juice
• 1/4 tsp salt
• 1/4 tsp black pepper
• 1 tbsp olive oil

Avocado Sauce:
• 1 ripe avocado, mashed
• 1/4 cup plain Greek yogurt
• 1 tbsp lemon juice
• 1 tbsp chopped fresh dill
• 1/4 tsp salt
• 1/4 tsp black pepper

Instructions:

1. In a medium bowl, combine the flaked salmon, beaten egg, almond flour, chopped parsley, lemon juice, salt, and pepper. Mix well until fully incorporated.

2. Form the salmon mixture into 4•6 patties, about 1/2 inch thick.

3. In a large skillet, heat the olive oil over medium heat. Carefully add the salmon cakes and cook for 3•4 minutes per side, until golden brown.

4. While the salmon cakes are cooking, make the avocado sauce. In a small bowl, mash the avocado and mix in the Greek yogurt, lemon juice, chopped dill, salt, and pepper.

5. Serve the warm salmon cakes topped with the creamy avocado sauce.

This Salmon Cakes with Avocado Sauce dish is an excellent choice for the Galveston Diet and menopausal women. Salmon is a rich source of omega•3 fatty acids, which can help reduce inflammation and support heart health. The avocado sauce provides a creamy, nutrient•dense topping that is high in healthy fats and antioxidants.

The almond flour in the salmon cakes helps to keep the dish low in carbs, while the egg and Greek yogurt provide a good source of protein. The fresh herbs and lemon juice add flavor without the need for excessive sodium or sugar.

This recipe is easy to prepare and can be enjoyed as a main course or a light meal. It's a versatile and nutritious option that can be customized to your personal taste preferences. The Salmon Cakes with Avocado Sauce are a great way to incorporate more heart•healthy, anti•inflammatory foods into your diet during menopause.

43. Southwest Quinoa Salad

Ingredient:

• 1 cup cooked quinoa, cooled
• 1 (15 oz) can black beans, rinsed and drained
• 1 cup diced bell pepper (any color)
• 1/2 cup diced red onion
• 1/2 cup corn kernels (fresh or frozen)
• 1/4 cup chopped cilantro
• 2 tbsp lime juice
• 1 tbsp olive oil
• 1 tsp ground cumin
• 1/4 tsp chili powder
• 1/4 tsp salt
• 1/4 tsp black pepper

Instructions:

1. In a large bowl, combine the cooked and cooled quinoa, rinsed black beans, diced bell pepper, diced red onion, corn kernels, and chopped cilantro.

2. In a small bowl, whisk together the lime juice, olive oil, cumin, chili powder, salt, and black pepper.

3. Pour the dressing over the quinoa salad and toss gently to coat.

4. Cover and refrigerate the Southwest Quinoa Salad for at least 30 minutes to allow the flavors to meld. Serve chilled or at room temperature.

This Southwest Quinoa Salad is an excellent choice for the Galveston Diet and menopausal women. Quinoa is a high•protein, gluten•free grain that is rich in fiber, vitamins, and minerals. The black beans, bell peppers, and corn provide additional fiber, vitamins, and antioxidants.

The combination of lime juice, olive oil, cumin, and chili powder creates a flavorful, zesty dressing that complements the other ingredients without the need for excessive sodium or sugar.

This salad is easy to prepare and can be made in advance, making it a convenient and nutritious option for busy menopausal women. It can be enjoyed as a main dish or a side, and it's a great way to incorporate more plant•based, low•carb foods into your diet during menopause.

44. Grilled Chicken with Peach Salsa

Ingredient:

Peach Salsa:
- 2 ripe peaches, diced
- 1/2 red onion, finely chopped
- 1 jalapeño, seeded and finely chopped
- 2 tbsp chopped fresh cilantro
- 1 tbsp lime juice
- 1/4 tsp salt

Grilled Chicken:
- 4 boneless, skinless chicken breasts
- 1 tbsp olive oil
- 1 tsp garlic powder
- 1 tsp paprika
- 1/2 tsp salt
- 1/4 tsp black pepper

Instructions:

1. Make the peach salsa: In a medium bowl, combine the diced peaches, chopped red onion, seeded and chopped jalapeño, chopped cilantro, lime juice, and salt. Stir to mix well and set aside.

2. Prepare the grilled chicken: Preheat your grill or grill pan to medium•high heat.

3. Pat the chicken breasts dry and brush them with the olive oil. Season both sides with the garlic powder, paprika, salt, and black pepper.

4. Grill the chicken for 5•7 minutes per side, or until it reaches an internal temperature of 165°F.

5. Transfer the grilled chicken to a serving platter and top with the fresh peach salsa. Serve the Grilled Chicken with Peach Salsa immediately.

This dish is an excellent choice for the Galveston Diet and menopausal women. Chicken is a lean protein that is low in calories and high in nutrients, while the peach salsa provides a sweet and tangy contrast that is rich in vitamins, minerals, and antioxidants.

The combination of the grilled chicken and the peach salsa is not only delicious but also nutritious. The healthy fats from the olive oil and the fiber from the peaches and onions can help support overall health during menopause.

This recipe is easy to prepare and can be enjoyed as a main course or a side dish. It's a versatile and flavorful option that can be customized to your personal taste preferences. The Grilled Chicken with Peach Salsa is a great way to incorporate more nutrient•dense, low•carb foods into your diet during menopause.

45. Eggplant Caponata

Ingredient:

- 1 medium eggplant, diced into 1·inch cubes
- 2 tbsp olive oil
- 1 onion, diced
- 3 cloves garlic, minced
- 1 (14 oz) can diced tomatoes
- 2 tbsp red wine vinegar
- 2 tbsp capers, rinsed and drained
- 1/4 cup pitted and chopped kalamata olives
- 2 tbsp chopped fresh basil
- 1 tsp dried oregano
- 1/4 tsp red pepper flakes (optional)
- Salt and pepper to taste

Instructions:

1. In a large skillet, heat the olive oil over medium·high heat. Add the diced eggplant and sauté for 5·7 minutes, until the eggplant is starting to soften.

2. Add the diced onion and minced garlic to the skillet. Cook for 2·3 minutes, until the onion is translucent.

3. Stir in the diced tomatoes, red wine vinegar, capers, chopped olives, fresh basil, dried oregano, and red pepper flakes (if using). Season with salt and pepper to taste.

4. Reduce the heat to medium·low and let the caponata simmer for 15·20 minutes, stirring occasionally, until the flavors have melded and the eggplant is very soft.

5. Serve the Eggplant Caponata warm or at room temperature, as a side dish or appetizer. It can also be served over grilled or roasted meats, fish, or as a topping for crostini.

This Eggplant Caponata is a delicious and nutritious dish that is suitable for the Galveston Diet and menopausal women. Eggplant is a low·carb, fiber·rich vegetable that is packed with antioxidants and vitamins. The combination of tomatoes, olives, capers, and herbs provides a flavorful, Mediterranean·inspired taste.

The healthy fats from the olive oil and the fiber from the vegetables make this caponata a satisfying and satiating option. It's also low in sodium and free from added sugars, making it a great choice for managing blood sugar levels and supporting overall health during menopause.

This recipe is easy to prepare and can be made in advance, making it a convenient and nutritious option for busy menopausal women. Enjoy the Eggplant Caponata as a side dish, appetizer, or topping for a variety of meals.

46. Berry Smoothie Bowl

Ingredient:

• 1 cup frozen mixed berries (such as blueberries, raspberries, and blackberries)
• 1/2 cup unsweetened almond milk
• 1/4 cup plain Greek yogurt
• 1 tbsp chia seeds
• 1 tbsp almond butter
• 1 tsp honey (optional)

Toppings:
• Fresh berries
• Sliced almonds
• Unsweetened coconut flakes
• Mint leaves

Instructions:

1. In a high•speed blender, combine the frozen mixed berries, almond milk, Greek yogurt, chia seeds, and almond butter. Blend until smooth and creamy.

2. If desired, add the honey and blend again briefly to incorporate.

3. Pour the smoothie into a bowl. Top the smoothie bowl with the fresh berries, sliced almonds, unsweetened coconut flakes, and mint leaves.

This Berry Smoothie Bowl is an excellent choice for the Galveston Diet and menopausal women. It's packed with nutrient•dense ingredients that can help support overall health during menopause.

The frozen berries provide a good source of antioxidants, fiber, and vitamins. The Greek yogurt adds protein and probiotics, while the almond milk and almond butter contribute healthy fats. The chia seeds are a great source of fiber, protein, and omega•3 fatty acids.

The toppings not only add texture and visual appeal but also provide additional nutrients and healthy fats. The fresh berries, sliced almonds, and coconut flakes complement the flavors of the smoothie and make this a satisfying and nutritious meal or snack.

This Berry Smoothie Bowl is easy to prepare and can be enjoyed for breakfast, lunch, or as a healthy treat. It's a versatile and nutrient•dense option that can be customized to your personal taste preferences.

47. Cabbage Stir•Fry with Chicken

Ingredient:

• 1 lb boneless, skinless chicken breasts, cut into 1•inch pieces
• 2 tbsp sesame oil
• 4 cups shredded green cabbage
• 1 cup shredded red cabbage
• 1 red bell pepper, sliced
• 3 cloves garlic, minced
• 1 tbsp grated fresh ginger
• 2 tbsp low•sodium soy sauce
• 1 tbsp rice vinegar
• 1 tsp sesame seeds
• Salt and pepper to taste

Instructions:

1. In a large skillet or wok, heat the sesame oil over medium•high heat.

2. Add the cubed chicken and stir•fry for 5•7 minutes, until the chicken is cooked through and no longer pink.

3. Add the shredded green and red cabbage, sliced red bell pepper, minced garlic, and grated ginger to the skillet. Stir•fry for 5•7 minutes, until the vegetables are tender•crisp.

4. Stir in the soy sauce and rice vinegar, and toss to coat the vegetables and chicken.

5. Remove the skillet from heat and sprinkle the sesame seeds over the top. Season the Cabbage Stir•Fry with Chicken with salt and pepper to taste. Serve the stir•fry immediately, while hot.

This Cabbage Stir•Fry with Chicken is an excellent choice for the Galveston Diet and menopausal women. Cabbage is a low•carb, nutrient•dense vegetable that is rich in fiber, vitamins, and antioxidants, which can help support overall health during menopause.

The addition of chicken provides a lean protein source, while the sesame oil, soy sauce, and rice vinegar add flavor without the need for excessive sodium or sugar. The ginger and garlic also provide a flavorful boost and potential anti•inflammatory benefits.

This recipe is easy to prepare and can be made in a single skillet or wok, making it a convenient and nutritious option for busy menopausal women. The Cabbage Stir•Fry with Chicken can be enjoyed as a main dish or a side, and it's a great way to incorporate more low•carb, plant•based foods into your diet.

48. Sweet Potato and Black Bean Enchiladas

Ingredient:

• 2 medium sweet potatoes, peeled and diced
• 1 tablespoon olive oil
• 1 onion, diced
• 3 cloves garlic, minced
• 1 (15 oz) can black beans, drained and rinsed
• 1 teaspoon ground cumin
• 1 teaspoon chili powder
• 1/2 teaspoon smoked paprika
• Salt and pepper to taste
• 12 corn tortillas
• 1 (15 oz) can enchilada sauce
• 1 cup shredded Mexican cheese blend

Instructions:

1. Preheat oven to 375°F. Grease a 9x13 inch baking dish.

2. In a large skillet, heat the olive oil over medium heat. Add the diced sweet potatoes and sauté for 8•10 minutes until tender.

3. Add the onion and garlic to the skillet and cook for 2•3 minutes until fragrant.

4. Stir in the black beans, cumin, chili powder, smoked paprika, salt and pepper. Cook for 2•3 minutes more.

5. Spread 1/2 cup of the enchilada sauce in the bottom of the prepared baking dish.

6. Spoon about 1/4 cup of the sweet potato and black bean mixture onto each tortilla. Roll up the tortillas and place seam•side down in the baking dish.

7. Pour the remaining enchilada sauce over the top of the rolled enchiladas. Sprinkle with the shredded cheese.

8. Bake for 20•25 minutes until heated through and the cheese is melted.

9. Serve hot, garnished with chopped cilantro, diced avocado, or sour cream if desired.

Enjoy your homemade sweet potato and black bean enchiladas!

49. Spinach and Mushroom Quiche

Ingredient:

- 1 pre•made whole wheat pie crust
- 8 oz fresh spinach, chopped
- 8 oz sliced mushrooms
- 1 small onion, diced
- 3 large eggs
- 1 cup unsweetened almond milk
- 1/2 cup crumbled feta cheese
- 1 tsp dried thyme
- 1/2 tsp salt
- 1/4 tsp black pepper

Instructions:

1. Preheat oven to 375°F. Prepare the pie crust in a 9•inch pie dish.

2. In a skillet over medium heat, sauté the mushrooms and onion for 5•7 minutes until softened.

3. Add the chopped spinach and cook for 2•3 minutes until wilted. Remove from heat and let cool slightly.

4. In a medium bowl, whisk together the eggs and almond milk. Stir in the feta cheese, thyme, salt and pepper.

5. Spread the spinach and mushroom mixture evenly in the prepared pie crust. Pour the egg mixture over top.

6. Bake for 35•40 minutes, until the center is set. Allow to cool for 10 minutes before slicing and serving.

This quiche is a great option for the Galveston Diet as it is high in protein, low in carbs, and contains beneficial nutrients like spinach and mushrooms. The feta cheese also provides calcium which is important during menopause. Enjoy!

50. Grilled Steak Salad with Blue Cheese Dressing

Ingredient:

Salad:

- 1 lb flank steak
- 8 cups mixed greens
- 1 cup cherry tomatoes, halved
- 1/2 cup sliced cucumber
- 1/4 cup crumbled blue cheese

Blue Cheese Dressing:

- 1/2 cup plain Greek yogurt
- 2 tbsp crumbled blue cheese
- 1 tbsp lemon juice
- 1 tsp Dijon mustard
- 1 clove garlic, minced
- 1/4 tsp salt
- 1/4 tsp black pepper

Instructions:

1. Preheat your grill or grill pan to medium•high heat.

2. Season the flank steak with salt and pepper. Grill the steak for 4•6 minutes per side, or until it reaches your desired doneness. Let the steak rest for 5 minutes, then slice it against the grain.

3. In a large salad bowl, combine the mixed greens, halved cherry tomatoes, and sliced cucumber.

4. In a small bowl, whisk together the ingredients for the blue cheese dressing: Greek yogurt, crumbled blue cheese, lemon juice, Dijon mustard, minced garlic, salt, and black pepper.

5. Add the sliced grilled steak to the salad bowl. Drizzle the blue cheese dressing over the top and toss gently to coat. Sprinkle the additional crumbled blue cheese over the salad. Serve the Grilled Steak Salad with Blue Cheese Dressing immediately.

This Grilled Steak Salad is an excellent choice for the Galveston Diet and menopausal women. Flank steak is a lean, high•protein cut of beef that is rich in nutrients, while the mixed greens, tomatoes, and cucumber provide a variety of vitamins, minerals, and antioxidants.

The blue cheese dressing is made with healthy fats from the Greek yogurt and blue cheese, and it adds a creamy, tangy flavor to the salad without the need for excessive sodium or sugar.

This recipe is easy to prepare and can be enjoyed as a main dish or a side. It's a versatile and nutritious option that can be customized to your personal taste preferences. The Grilled Steak Salad with Blue Cheese Dressing is a great way to incorporate more lean protein, healthy fats, and nutrient•dense vegetables into your diet during menopause.

51. Lemon Herb Roasted Chicken

Ingredient:

- 1 (3•4 lb) whole chicken
- 2 tbsp olive oil
- 2 tbsp lemon juice
- 2 tsp dried thyme
- 2 tsp dried rosemary
- 1 tsp garlic powder
- 1 tsp salt
- 1/2 tsp black pepper

Instructions:

1. Preheat oven to 400°F. Pat the chicken dry with paper towels.

2. In a small bowl, mix together the olive oil, lemon juice, thyme, rosemary, garlic powder, salt and pepper.

3. Rub the seasoning mixture all over the outside of the chicken, making sure to get it under the skin as well.

4. Place the chicken in a roasting pan or baking dish. Roast for 60•75 minutes, until the internal temperature reaches 165°F.

5. Let the chicken rest for 10 minutes before carving and serving.

This lemon herb roasted chicken is a great option for the Galveston Diet. It's high in protein, low in carbs, and the herbs and lemon provide beneficial antioxidants. The healthy fats from the olive oil also help promote satiety.

Chicken is an excellent source of lean protein, which is important during menopause to help maintain muscle mass. The herbs and lemon add flavor without the need for heavy sauces or seasonings.

Serve this chicken with roasted vegetables or a fresh salad for a complete, nutrient•dense meal. Enjoy!

52. Ratatouille Stuffed Bell Peppers

Ingredient:

- 4 large bell peppers, halved and seeded
- 1 tbsp olive oil
- 1 medium eggplant, diced
- 1 zucchini, diced
- 1 yellow squash, diced
- 1 onion, diced
- 3 cloves garlic, minced
- 1 (14.5 oz) can diced tomatoes
- 2 tsp dried basil
- 1 tsp dried oregano
- 1/2 tsp salt
- 1/4 tsp black pepper
- 1/2 cup crumbled feta cheese

Instructions:

1. Preheat oven to 375°F. Place the bell pepper halves in a baking dish and set aside.

2. In a large skillet, heat the olive oil over medium heat. Add the eggplant, zucchini, squash, onion and garlic. Sauté for 8•10 minutes until vegetables are tender.

3. Stir in the diced tomatoes, basil, oregano, salt and pepper. Simmer for 5 minutes.

4. Spoon the ratatouille mixture evenly into the bell pepper halves. Top with the crumbled feta cheese.

5. Bake for 25•30 minutes, until the peppers are tender.

6. Serve hot, garnished with fresh basil if desired.

These ratatouille stuffed peppers are a great option for the Galveston Diet. They are low in carbs, high in fiber and antioxidants from the vegetables, and provide a good source of protein from the feta cheese. The healthy fats from the olive oil also help promote satiety.

The vegetables and herbs make this a nutrient•dense meal that is suitable for menopause. The bell peppers provide vitamin C, which can help support immune function during this time.

53. Asparagus and Goat Cheese Frittata

Ingredient:

• 1 lb asparagus, trimmed and cut into 1•inch pieces
• 8 large eggs
• 2 oz crumbled goat cheese
• 2 tbsp olive oil
• 1 shallot, minced
• 2 cloves garlic, minced
• Salt and pepper to taste

Instructions:

1. Preheat oven to 375°F.

2. In a 9•inch oven•safe nonstick skillet, heat the olive oil over medium heat. Add the asparagus, shallot, and garlic. Sauté for 5•7 minutes until the asparagus is tender.

3. In a bowl, whisk the eggs. Season with salt and pepper.

4. Pour the egg mixture over the asparagus in the skillet. Sprinkle the crumbled goat cheese over the top.

5. Transfer the skillet to the oven and bake for 15•18 minutes, until the eggs are set.

6. Allow to cool for 5 minutes, then slice and serve.

This frittata is a great source of protein, fiber, and healthy fats from the asparagus, eggs, and goat cheese. It's a nutritious and satisfying meal that fits well within the guidelines of the Galveston Diet for women during menopause.

54. Chickpea and Vegetable Tagine

Ingredient:

- 1 tbsp olive oil
- 1 onion, diced
- 3 cloves garlic, minced
- 1 tsp ground cumin
- 1 tsp ground coriander
- 1 tsp paprika
- 1/2 tsp ground cinnamon
- 1/4 tsp cayenne pepper (or to taste)
- 1 (15 oz) can chickpeas, drained and rinsed
- 1 (14 oz) can diced tomatoes
- 1 cup vegetable broth
- 1 medium eggplant, diced
- 1 medium zucchini, diced
- 1 red bell pepper, diced
- 2 tbsp chopped fresh parsley
- Salt and pepper to taste

Instructions:

1. In a large pot or Dutch oven, heat the olive oil over medium heat. Add the diced onion and sauté for 3·4 minutes, until translucent.

2. Add the minced garlic, cumin, coriander, paprika, cinnamon, and cayenne pepper. Cook for 1 minute, until fragrant.

3. Stir in the drained and rinsed chickpeas, diced tomatoes, and vegetable broth. Bring the mixture to a simmer.

4. Add the diced eggplant, zucchini, and red bell pepper to the pot. Reduce the heat to medium·low and let the tagine simmer for 20·25 minutes, until the vegetables are tender.

5. Remove the pot from heat and stir in the chopped fresh parsley. Season with salt and pepper to taste. Serve the Chickpea and Vegetable Tagine warm, over cauliflower rice or with a side of roasted vegetables.

This Chickpea and Vegetable Tagine is an excellent choice for the Galveston Diet and menopausal women. Chickpeas are a good source of plant·based protein, fiber, and complex carbohydrates, while the vegetables provide a variety of vitamins, minerals, and antioxidants.

The blend of spices, including cumin, coriander, paprika, and cinnamon, adds a flavorful, aromatic depth to the dish without the need for excessive sodium or sugar. The cayenne pepper provides a subtle heat that can help alleviate some menopausal symptoms.

This recipe is easy to prepare and can be made in a single pot, making it a convenient and nutritious option for busy menopausal women. The Chickpea and Vegetable Tagine can be enjoyed as a main dish or a side, and it's a great way to incorporate more plant·based, low·carb foods into your diet.

55. Kale and Quinoa Salad with Lemon Vinaigrette

Ingredient:

Salad:
• 4 cups chopped kale, stems removed
• 1 cup cooked quinoa, cooled
• 1/2 cup diced cucumber
• 1/4 cup crumbled feta cheese
• 2 tbsp toasted sliced almonds

Lemon Vinaigrette:
• 2 tbsp olive oil
• 2 tbsp lemon juice
• 1 tsp Dijon mustard
• 1 tsp honey
• 1/4 tsp salt
• 1/4 tsp black pepper

Instructions:

1. In a large bowl, combine the chopped kale, cooked quinoa, diced cucumber, crumbled feta cheese, and toasted sliced almonds.

2. In a small bowl, whisk together the olive oil, lemon juice, Dijon mustard, honey, salt, and black pepper to make the lemon vinaigrette.

3. Pour the lemon vinaigrette over the kale and quinoa salad and toss gently to coat.

4. Let the salad sit for 5•10 minutes to allow the flavors to meld.

5. Serve the Kale and Quinoa Salad chilled or at room temperature.

This Kale and Quinoa Salad with Lemon Vinaigrette is an excellent choice for the Galveston Diet and menopausal women. Kale is a nutrient•dense leafy green that is high in fiber, vitamins, and antioxidants, which can help support overall health during menopause.

The quinoa provides a good source of plant•based protein and complex carbohydrates, while the feta cheese and toasted almonds add healthy fats and a creamy, crunchy texture.

The lemon vinaigrette dressing is made with healthy fats from the olive oil and a touch of honey for sweetness, without any added sugars. The Dijon mustard and lemon juice provide a tangy, flavorful contrast to the other ingredients.

This salad is easy to prepare and can be made in advance, making it a convenient and nutritious option for busy menopausal women. It can be enjoyed as a main dish or a side, and it's a great way to incorporate more plant•based, low•carb foods into your diet.

56. Baked Stuffed Zucchini Boats

Ingredient:

- 4 medium zucchini, halved lengthwise
- 1 lb ground turkey or lean ground beef
- 1 cup cooked quinoa
- 1/2 cup diced onion
- 2 cloves garlic, minced
- 1 tsp dried oregano
- 1/2 tsp dried basil
- 1/4 tsp red pepper flakes (optional)
- 1 cup marinara sauce
- 1/2 cup shredded mozzarella cheese

Lemon Vinaigrette:
- 2 tbsp olive oil
- 2 tbsp lemon juice
- 1 tsp Dijon mustard
- 1 tsp honey
- 1/4 tsp salt
- 1/4 tsp black pepper

Instructions:

1. Preheat oven to 375°F.

2. Scoop out the flesh from the zucchini halves, leaving about 1/4 inch of the zucchini shell. Finely chop the scooped•out zucchini flesh.

3. In a skillet over medium heat, cook the ground turkey or beef until browned and crumbled, 5•7 minutes. Drain any excess fat.

4. Add the chopped zucchini flesh, onion, garlic, oregano, basil, and red pepper flakes (if using) to the skillet. Sauté for 3•4 minutes until the vegetables are tender.

5. Stir in the cooked quinoa and 1/2 cup of the marinara sauce. Season with salt and pepper to taste.

6. Arrange the zucchini boats in a baking dish. Spoon the filling into the zucchini shells, packing it in tightly.

7. Top each stuffed zucchini boat with the remaining 1/2 cup of marinara sauce and the shredded mozzarella cheese.

8. Bake for 20•25 minutes, until the zucchini is tender and the cheese is melted and bubbly. Serve hot.

These Baked Stuffed Zucchini Boats are a great source of fiber, protein, and nutrients that are beneficial during menopause. The combination of zucchini, quinoa, and lean protein makes this a satisfying and healthy meal that fits well within the Galveston Diet guidelines.

57. Teriyaki Tofu Stir•Fry

Ingredient:

• 1 block (14 oz) extra•firm tofu, pressed and cubed
• 2 tbsp sesame oil
• 1 cup broccoli florets
• 1 red bell pepper, sliced
• 1 cup sliced mushrooms
• 2 cloves garlic, minced
• 1 tbsp grated fresh ginger
• 1/4 cup low•sodium teriyaki sauce
• 2 tsp sesame seeds
• Salt and pepper to taste

Instructions:

1. In a large skillet or wok, heat the sesame oil over medium•high heat.

2. Add the cubed tofu and cook for 5•7 minutes, turning occasionally, until lightly browned on all sides. Remove tofu from the pan and set aside.

3. Add the broccoli, bell pepper, mushrooms, garlic, and ginger to the pan. Stir•fry for 5•7 minutes until the vegetables are tender•crisp.

4. Return the tofu to the pan and pour in the teriyaki sauce. Toss everything together and cook for 2•3 minutes until the sauce thickens slightly.

5. Remove from heat and sprinkle with sesame seeds. Season with salt and pepper to taste. Serve immediately over steamed brown rice or quinoa.

This Teriyaki Tofu Stir•Fry is a great source of plant•based protein, fiber, and antioxidants. The vegetables and tofu provide a variety of nutrients that are beneficial during menopause, while the teriyaki sauce adds a delicious flavor. It's a quick and easy meal that fits well within the Galveston Diet guidelines.

58. Mediterranean Tuna Salad

Ingredient:

• 2 (5 oz) cans of tuna, drained and flaked
• 1/2 cup diced cucumber
• 1/2 cup diced tomatoes
• 1/4 cup diced red onion
• 2 tbsp chopped kalamata olives
• 2 tbsp crumbled feta cheese
• 2 tbsp chopped fresh parsley
• 2 tbsp olive oil
• 1 tbsp red wine vinegar
• 1 tsp Dijon mustard
• 1 tsp dried oregano
• Salt and pepper to taste

Instructions:

1. In a large bowl, combine the flaked tuna, cucumber, tomatoes, red onion, kalamata olives, feta cheese, and parsley.

2. In a small bowl, whisk together the olive oil, red wine vinegar, Dijon mustard, and dried oregano. Season with salt and pepper.

3. Pour the dressing over the tuna and vegetable mixture and toss gently to coat.

4. Serve the Mediterranean Tuna Salad on a bed of mixed greens or stuffed into tomatoes or avocado halves.

This Mediterranean Tuna Salad is a great option for the Galveston Diet during menopause. The tuna provides lean protein, while the vegetables, olives, and feta cheese add fiber, healthy fats, and antioxidants. The olive oil and vinegar dressing is a flavorful and heart•healthy way to dress the salad.

This dish can be enjoyed on its own or served with whole grain crackers or a side of roasted vegetables for a complete and satisfying meal.

59. Grilled Vegetable Skewers with Chimichurri Sauce

Ingredient:

Vegetable Skewers:
• 1 zucchini, cut into 1•inch pieces
• 1 yellow squash, cut into 1•inch pieces
• 1 red bell pepper, cut into 1•inch pieces
• 1 red onion, cut into 1•inch pieces
• 8 oz cremini mushrooms, halved
• 2 tbsp olive oil
• Salt and pepper to taste

Chimichurri Sauce:
• 1 cup packed fresh parsley leaves
• 3 cloves garlic
• 2 tbsp red wine vinegar
• 1 tbsp olive oil
• 1 tsp dried oregano
• 1/4 tsp red pepper flakes
• Salt and pepper to taste

Instructions:

1. Preheat grill to medium•high heat.

2. Thread the prepared vegetables onto skewers, leaving a little space between each piece.

3. Brush the skewers with the 2 tbsp of olive oil and season with salt and pepper.

4. Grill the vegetable skewers for 12•15 minutes, turning occasionally, until the vegetables are tender and lightly charred.

5. While the skewers are grilling, make the chimichurri sauce. In a food processor, combine the parsley, garlic, vinegar, 1 tbsp olive oil, oregano, and red pepper flakes. Pulse until a coarse paste forms. Season with salt and pepper to taste.

6. Serve the grilled vegetable skewers warm, drizzled with the chimichurri sauce.

This Grilled Vegetable Skewers with Chimichurri Sauce dish is a great option for the Galveston Diet during menopause. The variety of vegetables provide fiber, vitamins, and antioxidants, while the chimichurri sauce adds a flavorful punch of herbs and spices. The healthy fats from the olive oil and the anti•inflammatory properties of the herbs make this a nutritious and satisfying meal.

60. Sesame Ginger Baked Salmon

Ingredient:

• 4 (6 oz) salmon fillets
• 2 tbsp low•sodium soy sauce
• 1 tbsp rice vinegar
• 1 tbsp sesame oil
• 1 tbsp honey
• 1 tbsp grated fresh ginger
• 2 cloves garlic, minced
• 1 tsp sesame seeds
• Salt and pepper to taste

Instructions:

1. Preheat oven to 400°F.

2. In a small bowl, whisk together the soy sauce, rice vinegar, sesame oil, honey, grated ginger, and minced garlic.

3. Place the salmon fillets in a baking dish and season with salt and pepper.

4. Pour the soy sauce mixture over the salmon, making sure to coat the fillets evenly.

5. Sprinkle the sesame seeds over the top of the salmon.

6. Bake for 12•15 minutes, or until the salmon is cooked through and flakes easily with a fork.

7. Serve the Sesame Ginger Baked Salmon immediately, garnished with additional sesame seeds if desired.

This Sesame Ginger Baked Salmon is a delicious and nutritious option for the Galveston Diet during menopause. Salmon is an excellent source of omega•3 fatty acids, which are beneficial for heart health and reducing inflammation. The ginger, garlic, and sesame flavors add a flavorful Asian•inspired twist to the dish.

Serve the salmon with a side of roasted vegetables or a fresh salad for a complete and balanced meal. This recipe is easy to prepare and is sure to become a new favorite.

61. Roasted Beet and Arugula Salad with Walnuts

Ingredient:

• 3 medium beets, peeled and cut into 1•inch cubes
• 2 tbsp olive oil
• Salt and pepper to taste
• 5 oz baby arugula
• 1/4 cup crumbled feta cheese
• 1/4 cup chopped walnuts
• 2 tbsp balsamic vinegar
• 1 tbsp Dijon mustard
• 1 tbsp honey

Instructions:

1. Preheat oven to 400°F.

2. Toss the cubed beets with 1 tbsp of the olive oil and season with salt and pepper.

3. Spread the beets on a baking sheet and roast for 20•25 minutes, until tender and lightly caramelized. Allow to cool slightly.

4. In a large salad bowl, combine the roasted beets, arugula, feta cheese, and walnuts.

5. In a small bowl, whisk together the remaining 1 tbsp olive oil, balsamic vinegar, Dijon mustard, and honey. Season with salt and pepper.

6. Drizzle the dressing over the salad and toss gently to coat. Serve immediately.

This Roasted Beet and Arugula Salad is a nutrient•dense and flavorful dish that is perfect for the Galveston Diet. The beets provide fiber, folate, and antioxidants, while the arugula is a great source of vitamins A, C, and K. The walnuts add healthy fats and crunch, and the feta cheese provides a creamy, tangy contrast. The balsamic vinaigrette ties all the flavors together.

This salad is a great way to incorporate a variety of beneficial nutrients into your diet during menopause.

62. Thai Peanut Zoodles

Ingredient:

- 3•4 medium zucchinis, spiralized into noodles (about 4 cups of zoodles)
- 1/4 cup creamy peanut butter
- 2 tablespoons low•sodium soy sauce
- 2 tablespoons lime juice
- 1 tablespoon honey
- 1 teaspoon sesame oil
- 1 garlic clove, minced
- 1/4 teaspoon red pepper flakes (optional)
- 2 tablespoons chopped fresh cilantro
- 2 tablespoons chopped roasted peanuts

Instructions:

1. In a medium bowl, whisk together the peanut butter, soy sauce, lime juice, honey, sesame oil, and garlic until well combined.

2. Add the spiralized zucchini noodles to the peanut sauce and toss to coat evenly.

3. Sprinkle the red pepper flakes (if using), chopped cilantro, and chopped peanuts over the top.

4. Serve immediately. The zoodles will release some moisture as they sit, so it's best to serve right away.

Enjoy your Thai Peanut Zoodles! The peanut sauce adds a delicious nutty and slightly sweet flavor to the fresh zucchini noodles. This is a healthy, low•carb alternative to traditional pasta dishes.

63. Stuffed Bell Peppers with Ground Turkey and Quinoa

Ingredient:

• 4 large bell peppers (any color)
• 1 lb ground turkey
• 1 cup cooked quinoa
• 1/2 cup diced onion
• 2 cloves garlic, minced
• 1 tsp dried oregano
• 1/2 tsp ground cumin
• 1/4 tsp red pepper flakes (optional)
• 1 cup marinara sauce
• 1/2 cup shredded mozzarella cheese

Instructions:

1. Preheat oven to 375°F.

2. Cut the tops off the bell peppers and remove the seeds and membranes. Place the peppers in a baking dish and set aside.

3. In a skillet over medium heat, cook the ground turkey until browned and crumbled, about 5•7 minutes. Drain any excess fat.

4. Add the onion and garlic to the skillet and sauté for 2•3 minutes until fragrant.

5. Stir in the cooked quinoa, oregano, cumin, and red pepper flakes (if using).
Season with salt and pepper to taste.

6. Spoon the turkey and quinoa mixture into the hollowed•out bell peppers, packing it in tightly. Pour the marinara sauce around the base of the peppers in the baking dish. Cover the dish with foil and bake for 25•30 minutes.

7. Remove the foil, sprinkle the mozzarella cheese over the tops of the peppers, and bake for an additional 10•15 minutes, until the peppers are tender and the cheese is melted. Serve the Stuffed Bell Peppers warm.

These Stuffed Bell Peppers are a great option for the Galveston Diet during menopause. The combination of ground turkey, quinoa, and vegetables provides a nutrient•dense and satisfying meal. The bell peppers are a good source of vitamins A and C, while the quinoa adds fiber and protein. This dish is easy to prepare and can be made ahead of time for a quick and healthy weeknight dinner.

64. Cauliflower Rice Sushi Rolls

Ingredient:

• 1 head of cauliflower, riced
• 1 tablespoon rice vinegar
• 1 teaspoon coconut aminos (or low•sodium soy sauce)
• 1/2 teaspoon sesame oil
• 1/4 teaspoon salt
• 1 avocado, sliced
• 1 cucumber, julienned
• 1 carrot, julienned
• Nori sheets

Instructions:

1. In a food processor, pulse the cauliflower florets until they resemble rice grains. Transfer the cauliflower rice to a bowl.

2. In a small bowl, whisk together the rice vinegar, coconut aminos, sesame oil, and salt. Pour this mixture over the cauliflower rice and stir to combine.

3. Lay a nori sheet shiny•side down on a bamboo sushi mat or clean surface. Spread about 1/2 cup of the cauliflower rice mixture evenly over the nori sheet, leaving a 1•inch border at the top.

4. Arrange a few slices of avocado, cucumber, and carrot in a line across the center of the rice.

5. Carefully roll up the nori sheet, using the bamboo mat to help you roll it tightly. Moisten the top edge with water to seal the roll.

6. Slice the roll into 6•8 pieces using a sharp knife. Serve immediately.

Tips:
• The Galveston Diet recommends avoiding soy sauce, so use coconut aminos instead.
• Avocado, cucumber, and carrot are all great veggie options for these sushi rolls.
• You can also try other fillings like cooked shrimp, crab meat, or tofu.

Enjoy these healthy and delicious Cauliflower Rice Sushi Rolls! They make a great snack or light meal during menopause.

65. Lemon Garlic Shrimp with Quinoa

Ingredient:

• 1 cup uncooked quinoa, rinsed
• 2 cups low·sodium chicken or vegetable broth
• 1 lb large shrimp, peeled and deveined
• 2 tablespoons olive oil
• 3 garlic cloves, minced
• 1 tablespoon lemon juice
• 1 teaspoon lemon zest
• 1/4 teaspoon red pepper flakes (optional)
• 2 tablespoons chopped fresh parsley
• Salt and pepper to taste

Instructions:

1. In a medium saucepan, combine the quinoa and broth. Bring to a boil, then reduce heat to low, cover and simmer for 15·20 minutes until quinoa is tender and liquid is absorbed. Fluff with a fork.

2. In a large skillet, heat the olive oil over medium·high heat. Add the garlic and sauté for 1 minute until fragrant.

3. Add the shrimp to the skillet and cook for 2·3 minutes per side, until the shrimp are opaque and cooked through.

4. Remove the skillet from heat and stir in the lemon juice, lemon zest, and red pepper flakes (if using). Season with salt and pepper to taste.

5. Serve the lemon garlic shrimp over the cooked quinoa. Garnish with chopped fresh parsley.

Tips:
• The Galveston Diet recommends using low·sodium broth to control sodium intake.
• Quinoa is a great whole grain option that is high in protein and fiber.
• Lemon and garlic add bright, flavorful notes without the need for heavy sauces.

This Lemon Garlic Shrimp with Quinoa makes a healthy, balanced meal that is suitable for the Galveston Diet during menopause. Enjoy!

66. Baked Chicken Parmesan with Zucchini Noodles

Ingredient:

• 4 boneless, skinless chicken breasts
• 1/2 cup whole wheat breadcrumbs
• 1/4 cup grated Parmesan cheese
• 1 teaspoon dried oregano
• 1/2 teaspoon garlic powder
• 1/4 teaspoon salt
• 1/4 teaspoon black pepper
• 1 egg, beaten
• 3•4 medium zucchinis, spiralized into noodles
• 1 cup marinara sauce (no•sugar•added)

Instructions:

1. Preheat oven to 400°F. Line a baking sheet with parchment paper.

2. In a shallow bowl, combine the breadcrumbs, Parmesan, oregano, garlic powder, salt, and pepper.

3. Dip the chicken breasts in the beaten egg, then coat them evenly with the breadcrumb mixture, pressing to adhere.

4. Place the breaded chicken on the prepared baking sheet. Bake for 25•30 minutes, until the chicken is cooked through and the breading is golden brown.

5. While the chicken is baking, spiralize the zucchinis into noodles.

6. In a large skillet, heat the marinara sauce over medium heat. Add the zucchini noodles and toss to coat, cooking for 2•3 minutes until the noodles are tender but still crisp.

7. Serve the baked chicken parmesan over the zucchini noodles. Enjoy!

Tips:
• The Galveston Diet recommends using whole wheat breadcrumbs and no•sugar•added marinara sauce.
• Zucchini noodles are a great low•carb alternative to traditional pasta.
• This dish is high in protein, fiber, and nutrients, making it a great option for menopause.

This Baked Chicken Parmesan with Zucchini Noodles is a delicious and healthy meal that fits perfectly within the Galveston Diet guidelines.

67. Quinoa Stuffed Acorn Squash

Ingredient:
• 2 acorn squash, halved and seeded
• 1 cup uncooked quinoa, rinsed
• 2 cups low•sodium vegetable or chicken broth
• 1 tablespoon olive oil
• 1 onion, diced
• 2 cloves garlic, minced
• 1 cup diced mushrooms
• 1 cup diced bell pepper
• 1 teaspoon dried thyme
• 1/4 teaspoon salt
• 1/4 teaspoon black pepper
• 2 tablespoons chopped fresh parsley

Instructions:
1. Preheat oven to 400°F. Place the acorn squash halves cut•side down on a baking sheet. Bake for 30•40 minutes, until tender when pierced with a fork.

2. In a medium saucepan, combine the quinoa and broth. Bring to a boil, then reduce heat to low, cover and simmer for 15•20 minutes until quinoa is tender and liquid is absorbed. Fluff with a fork.

3. In a skillet, heat the olive oil over medium heat. Add the onion and sauté for 3•4 minutes until translucent.

4. Add the garlic, mushrooms, and bell pepper to the skillet. Cook for 5•7 minutes, stirring occasionally, until the vegetables are tender.

5. Stir the cooked quinoa, thyme, salt, and pepper into the vegetable mixture. Scoop the quinoa stuffing into the baked acorn squash halves. Return the stuffed squash to the oven and bake for an additional 10•15 minutes. Garnish with chopped fresh parsley before serving.

Tips:
• The Galveston Diet recommends using low•sodium broth to control sodium intake.
• Quinoa is a great whole grain option that is high in protein and fiber.
• Acorn squash is a nutrient•dense winter squash that is suitable for the Galveston Diet.

This Quinoa Stuffed Acorn Squash makes a delicious and healthy meal that fits perfectly within the Galveston Diet guidelines during menopause.

68. Kale and White Bean Soup

Ingredient:

- 1 tablespoon olive oil
- 1 onion, diced
- 3 garlic cloves, minced
- 4 cups low•sodium chicken or vegetable broth
- 1 (15 oz) can no•salt•added white beans, rinsed and drained
- 1 (14.5 oz) can no•salt•added diced tomatoes
- 1 teaspoon dried thyme
- 1/2 teaspoon dried oregano
- 1/4 teaspoon red pepper flakes (optional)
- 4 cups chopped kale, stems removed
- Salt and pepper to taste

Instructions:

1. In a large pot or Dutch oven, heat the olive oil over medium heat. Add the onion and sauté for 3•4 minutes until translucent.

2. Add the garlic and sauté for 1 minute until fragrant.

3. Pour in the broth, white beans, diced tomatoes, thyme, oregano, and red pepper flakes (if using). Bring the soup to a simmer.

4. Add the chopped kale to the pot and cook for 5•7 minutes, until the kale is wilted and tender.

5. Season the soup with salt and pepper to taste.

6. Serve the Kale and White Bean Soup hot.

Tips:
- The Galveston Diet recommends using low•sodium broth and no•salt•added canned beans to control sodium intake.
- Kale is a nutrient•dense leafy green that is high in fiber, vitamins, and minerals.
- White beans provide plant•based protein and fiber, which are important during menopause.

This Kale and White Bean Soup is a comforting, nourishing meal that fits perfectly within the Galveston Diet guidelines. It's a great option for a healthy lunch or dinner during menopause.

69. Grilled Lamb Chops with Mint Pesto

Ingredient:

• 8 lamb chops (about 1•1.5 lbs)
• 2 tablespoons olive oil
• Salt and pepper to taste

For the Mint Pesto:
• 1 cup fresh mint leaves
• 2 tablespoons pine nuts
• 1 garlic clove
• 2 tablespoons olive oil
• 1 tablespoon lemon juice
• 1/4 teaspoon salt

Instructions:

1. Make the mint pesto: In a food processor, combine the mint leaves, pine nuts, garlic, olive oil, lemon juice, and salt. Pulse until a coarse pesto forms. Set aside.

2. Preheat grill or grill pan to medium•high heat.

3. Pat the lamb chops dry and brush both sides with olive oil. Season generously with salt and pepper.

4. Grill the lamb chops for 3•4 minutes per side, or until they reach your desired doneness.

5. Transfer the grilled lamb chops to a plate and let rest for 5 minutes.

6. Serve the lamb chops warm, drizzled with the mint pesto.

Tips:
• The Galveston Diet recommends using lean protein sources like lamb, which is high in iron and other nutrients.
• Mint pesto adds a bright, fresh flavor without the need for heavy sauces.
• Grilling the lamb chops gives them a nice char and smoky flavor.

This Grilled Lamb Chops with Mint Pesto dish is a delicious and healthy option that fits well within the Galveston Diet guidelines during menopause. Enjoy!

70. Caprese Stuffed Avocados

Ingredient:

• 4 ripe avocados, halved and pitted
• 8 oz fresh mozzarella cheese, diced
• 1 cup cherry tomatoes, halved
• 1/4 cup fresh basil leaves, chopped
• 2 tablespoons balsamic glaze
• Salt and pepper to taste

Instructions:

1. In a medium bowl, gently mix together the diced mozzarella, halved cherry tomatoes, and chopped basil leaves. Season with a pinch of salt and pepper.

2. Scoop the cheese and tomato mixture evenly into the pitted avocado halves.

3. Drizzle the balsamic glaze over the top of the stuffed avocados.

4. Serve immediately.

Tips:
• The Galveston Diet encourages the use of healthy fats like those found in avocados.

• Mozzarella cheese is a low•fat dairy option that fits well within the diet.

• Balsamic glaze provides a sweet and tangy flavor without the need for heavy dressings.

• This dish is refreshing, nutrient•dense, and easy to prepare.

These Caprese Stuffed Avocados make a great light lunch, snack, or appetizer that aligns with the Galveston Diet guidelines during menopause. The combination of creamy avocado, fresh mozzarella, juicy tomatoes, and fragrant basil is both delicious and satisfying.

71. Sweet Potato and Kale Hash

Ingredient:

- 2 medium sweet potatoes, peeled and diced
- 1 tablespoon olive oil
- 1 onion, diced
- 3 garlic cloves, minced
- 4 cups chopped kale, stems removed
- 1 teaspoon ground cumin
- 1/4 teaspoon cayenne pepper (optional)
- Salt and pepper to taste
- 2 eggs (optional)

Instructions:

1. In a large skillet, heat the olive oil over medium heat. Add the diced sweet potatoes and sauté for 8•10 minutes, stirring occasionally, until they start to soften.

2. Add the diced onion to the skillet and continue cooking for 3•4 minutes until the onion is translucent.

3. Stir in the minced garlic and chopped kale. Cook for 5•7 minutes, until the kale is wilted and tender.

4. Season the hash with cumin, cayenne pepper (if using), salt, and pepper. Stir to combine.

5. If desired, create two wells in the hash and crack the eggs into them. Cover the skillet and cook the eggs for 3•5 minutes, until the whites are set but the yolks are still runny. Serve the Sweet Potato and Kale Hash warm, with the eggs on top if using.

Tips:
- The Galveston Diet encourages the use of nutrient•dense vegetables like sweet potatoes and kale.
- Cumin and cayenne add warmth and flavor without the need for heavy sauces.
- The optional eggs provide additional protein to make this dish more filling and satisfying.

This Sweet Potato and Kale Hash is a delicious, one•pan meal that fits perfectly within the Galveston Diet guidelines during menopause. It's a great way to incorporate more vegetables and healthy fats into your diet.

72. Tofu and Broccoli Stir•Fry

Ingredient:

• 1 block (14 oz) extra•firm tofu, cubed
• 2 tablespoons coconut aminos (or low•sodium soy sauce)
• 1 tablespoon rice vinegar
• 1 teaspoon sesame oil
• 1 tablespoon olive oil
• 3 cups broccoli florets
• 2 garlic cloves, minced
• 1 tablespoon grated fresh ginger
• 1/4 teaspoon red pepper flakes (optional)
• 2 tablespoons chopped green onions
• Salt and pepper to taste

Instructions:

1. In a small bowl, whisk together the coconut aminos (or soy sauce), rice vinegar, and sesame oil. Set aside.

2. Heat the olive oil in a large skillet or wok over medium•high heat. Add the cubed tofu and cook for 5•7 minutes, turning occasionally, until lightly browned on all sides. Transfer the tofu to a plate.

3. Add the broccoli florets to the skillet and stir•fry for 3•4 minutes, until the broccoli is crisp•tender.

4. Push the broccoli to the sides of the skillet and add the minced garlic and grated ginger to the center. Cook for 1 minute, until fragrant.

5. Add the cooked tofu back to the skillet and pour in the coconut aminos mixture. Toss everything together and cook for 2•3 minutes, until the sauce has thickened slightly.

6. Remove from heat and stir in the red pepper flakes (if using) and chopped green onions. Season the stir•fry with salt and pepper to taste. Serve immediately over steamed cauliflower rice or quinoa.

Tips:
• The Galveston Diet recommends using coconut aminos instead of soy sauce to reduce sodium intake.
• Tofu is a great plant•based protein source that is suitable for the Galveston Diet.
• Broccoli is a nutrient•dense vegetable that provides fiber, vitamins, and minerals

73. Mediterranean Baked Cod

Ingredient:

• 4 (6 oz) cod fillets
• 2 tablespoons olive oil
• 2 tablespoons lemon juice
• 2 garlic cloves, minced
• 1 teaspoon dried oregano
• 1/2 teaspoon dried basil
• 1/4 teaspoon red pepper flakes (optional)
• 1 cup cherry tomatoes, halved
• 1/2 cup kalamata olives, pitted and halved
• 2 tablespoons crumbled feta cheese
• Salt and pepper to taste
• Chopped fresh parsley for garnish

Instructions:

1. Preheat your oven to 400°F. Lightly grease a baking dish or line it with parchment paper.

2. In a small bowl, whisk together the olive oil, lemon juice, garlic, oregano, basil, and red pepper flakes (if using).

3. Place the cod fillets in the prepared baking dish. Pour the olive oil mixture over the top, making sure to evenly coat the fish.

4. Scatter the cherry tomatoes and kalamata olives around the cod fillets.

5. Bake for 15•20 minutes, or until the cod is opaque and flakes easily with a fork.

6. Remove the baked cod from the oven and sprinkle the crumbled feta cheese over the top. Season with salt and pepper to taste. Garnish with chopped fresh parsley before serving.

Tips:
• The Galveston Diet encourages the use of lean protein sources like cod, which is high in omega•3 fatty acids.
• Mediterranean flavors like lemon, garlic, and herbs add plenty of flavor without the need for heavy sauces.
• Tomatoes, olives, and feta provide healthy fats and antioxidants.

74. Cucumber Avocado Soup

Ingredient:

• 2 large cucumbers, peeled and chopped
• 1 ripe avocado, pitted and peeled
• 1 cup unsweetened almond milk
• 1 tablespoon fresh lemon juice
• 1 garlic clove, minced
• 1/4 teaspoon ground cumin
• 1/4 teaspoon ground coriander
• Salt and pepper to taste
• Chopped fresh herbs (such as dill, chives, or cilantro) for garnish

Instructions:

1. In a high•speed blender or food processor, combine the chopped cucumbers, avocado, almond milk, lemon juice, garlic, cumin, and coriander. Blend until smooth and creamy.

2. Taste the soup and season with salt and pepper as needed.

3. Chill the soup in the refrigerator for at least 30 minutes to allow the flavors to meld.

4. Serve the chilled Cucumber Avocado Soup garnished with chopped fresh herbs.

Tips:
• The Galveston Diet encourages the use of healthy fats like those found in avocados.

• Unsweetened almond milk is a dairy•free, low•calorie option that works well in this recipe.

• Cucumbers and avocados provide a refreshing, cooling base for this soup.

• Spices like cumin and coriander add depth of flavor without the need for heavy cream or other high•calorie ingredients.

This Cucumber Avocado Soup is a light, nourishing, and flavorful dish that fits perfectly within the Galveston Diet guidelines during menopause. It makes a great starter or a light main course on a warm day.

75. Brussels Sprouts Caesar Salad

Ingredient:

- 1 lb Brussels sprouts, trimmed and shredded or thinly sliced
- 1/4 cup grated Parmesan cheese
- 2 tablespoons olive oil
- 2 tablespoons lemon juice
- 1 tablespoon Dijon mustard
- 1 garlic clove, minced
- 1/4 teaspoon Worcestershire sauce (optional)
- Salt and pepper to taste
- Chopped fresh parsley for garnish

Instructions:

1. In a large bowl, combine the shredded or sliced Brussels sprouts and grated Parmesan cheese.

2. In a small bowl, whisk together the olive oil, lemon juice, Dijon mustard, garlic, and Worcestershire sauce (if using). Season with salt and pepper to taste.

3. Pour the dressing over the Brussels sprouts and Parmesan, and toss to coat everything evenly.

4. Serve the Brussels Sprouts Caesar Salad immediately, garnished with chopped fresh parsley.

Tips:
• The Galveston Diet encourages the use of cruciferous vegetables like Brussels sprouts, which are high in fiber, vitamins, and antioxidants.

• Parmesan cheese provides a flavorful, low•fat dairy option for this salad.

• The lemon juice, Dijon mustard, and Worcestershire sauce (if using) create a tangy, Caesar•inspired dressing without the need for heavy cream or mayonnaise.

This Brussels Sprouts Caesar Salad is a delicious and nutritious way to incorporate more vegetables into your diet during menopause. It's a great option for a light lunch or a side dish.

76. Baked Garlic Herb Salmon

Ingredient:

• 4 (6 oz) salmon fillets
• 2 tablespoons olive oil
• 3 garlic cloves, minced
• 1 tablespoon chopped fresh parsley
• 1 tablespoon chopped fresh dill
• 1 teaspoon dried oregano
• 1/4 teaspoon red pepper flakes (optional)
• Salt and pepper to taste
• Lemon wedges for serving

Instructions:

1. Preheat your oven to 400°F. Line a baking sheet with parchment paper or foil.

2. In a small bowl, mix together the olive oil, minced garlic, chopped parsley, chopped dill, dried oregano, and red pepper flakes (if using).

3. Place the salmon fillets on the prepared baking sheet. Generously season the salmon with salt and pepper.

4. Spoon the garlic•herb mixture evenly over the top of the salmon fillets, making sure to coat them completely.

5. Bake the salmon for 12•15 minutes, or until it flakes easily with a fork and is cooked through.

6. Serve the Baked Garlic Herb Salmon immediately, with lemon wedges on the side.

Tips:
• The Galveston Diet encourages the use of fatty fish like salmon, which are high in omega•3 fatty acids.
• Fresh herbs like parsley and dill add flavor without the need for heavy sauces or seasonings.
• Red pepper flakes provide a subtle heat that can be omitted if desired.

This Baked Garlic Herb Salmon is a simple, flavorful, and healthy dish that fits perfectly within the Galveston Diet guidelines during menopause. Enjoy!

77. Spinach and Ricotta Stuffed Mushrooms

Ingredient:

• 12 large mushrooms, stems removed and finely chopped
• 1 tablespoon olive oil
• 1/2 cup part•skim ricotta cheese
• 1 cup fresh spinach, chopped
• 2 tablespoons grated Parmesan cheese
• 1 garlic clove, minced
• 1/4 teaspoon dried oregano
• Salt and pepper to taste

Instructions:

1. Preheat your oven to 375°F. Lightly grease a baking sheet or line it with parchment paper.

2. Remove the stems from the mushrooms and finely chop them.

3. In a skillet, heat the olive oil over medium heat. Add the chopped mushroom stems and sauté for 2•3 minutes until softened.

4. In a medium bowl, mix together the sautéed mushroom stems, ricotta cheese, chopped spinach, Parmesan cheese, minced garlic, and dried oregano. Season with salt and pepper to taste.

5. Spoon the spinach and ricotta mixture evenly into the mushroom caps, packing it in gently.

6. Arrange the stuffed mushrooms on the prepared baking sheet.

7. Bake for 12•15 minutes, or until the mushrooms are tender and the filling is heated through.

8. Serve the Spinach and Ricotta Stuffed Mushrooms warm.

Tips:
• The Galveston Diet encourages the use of low•fat dairy products like part•skim ricotta cheese.
• Spinach is a nutrient•dense vegetable that provides fiber, vitamins, and minerals.
• These stuffed mushrooms make a great appetizer or side dish during menopause.

78. Quinoa and Sweet Potato Cakes

Ingredient:

- 1 cup cooked quinoa
- 1 cup mashed sweet potato (about 1 medium sweet potato)
- 1 egg, beaten
- 2 tablespoons almond flour
- 1 teaspoon ground cumin
- 1/2 teaspoon garlic powder
- 1/4 teaspoon cayenne pepper (optional)
- Salt and pepper to taste
- 1 tablespoon olive oil

Instructions:

1. In a medium bowl, combine the cooked quinoa, mashed sweet potato, beaten egg, almond flour, cumin, garlic powder, and cayenne pepper (if using). Season with salt and pepper to taste. Mix well until fully incorporated.

2. Heat the olive oil in a large non•stick skillet over medium heat.

3. Scoop heaping tablespoons of the quinoa and sweet potato mixture and gently flatten them into patties. Working in batches, cook the cakes for 3•4 minutes per side, until golden brown.

4. Transfer the cooked quinoa and sweet potato cakes to a paper towel•lined plate.

5. Serve the cakes warm, garnished with additional toppings if desired, such as a dollop of plain Greek yogurt, chopped fresh herbs, or a drizzle of honey.

Tips:
• The Galveston Diet encourages the use of nutrient•dense ingredients like quinoa and sweet potatoes.

• Almond flour helps bind the cakes together without the need for traditional flour.

• Spices like cumin and cayenne add flavor without the use of high•sodium seasonings. These cakes can be served as a main dish, side, or appetizer during menopause.

These Quinoa and Sweet Potato Cakes are a delicious, healthy, and versatile option that fits well within the Galveston Diet guidelines.

79. Chicken and Vegetable Lettuce Wraps

Ingredient:

- 1 lb boneless, skinless chicken breasts, diced
- 1 tablespoon olive oil
- 1 red bell pepper, diced
- 1 cup shredded carrots
- 1 cup sliced mushrooms
- 2 garlic cloves, minced
- 1 tablespoon low•sodium soy sauce or coconut aminos
- 1 teaspoon sesame oil
- 1/4 teaspoon ground ginger
- Salt and pepper to taste
- 12•16 large lettuce leaves (such as romaine or bibb)
- Chopped green onions and toasted sesame seeds for garnish (optional)

Instructions:

1. In a large skillet or wok, heat the olive oil over medium•high heat. Add the diced chicken and cook for 5•7 minutes, until no longer pink.

2. Add the diced bell pepper, shredded carrots, sliced mushrooms, and minced garlic to the skillet. Sauté for 3•4 minutes, until the vegetables are tender.

3. Stir in the soy sauce (or coconut aminos), sesame oil, and ground ginger. Season with salt and pepper to taste.

4. Spoon the chicken and vegetable mixture into the lettuce leaves.

5. Garnish the lettuce wraps with chopped green onions and toasted sesame seeds, if desired. Serve the Chicken and Vegetable Lettuce Wraps immediately.

Tips:
- The Galveston Diet recommends using low•sodium soy sauce or coconut aminos to control sodium intake.
- Lettuce leaves provide a low•carb, crunchy base for the flavorful chicken and vegetable filling.
- This dish is a great source of lean protein, vegetables, and healthy fats.

These Chicken and Vegetable Lettuce Wraps are a delicious, nutrient•dense, and easy•to•prepare meal that fits perfectly within the Galveston Diet guidelines during menopause.

80. Eggplant Rollatini with Marinara

Ingredient:

- 1 medium eggplant, sliced lengthwise into 1/4•inch thick slices
- 1 tablespoon olive oil
- 1 cup part•skim ricotta cheese
- 1/4 cup grated Parmesan cheese
- 1 egg, beaten
- 2 tablespoons chopped fresh basil
- 1 garlic clove, minced
- Salt and pepper to taste
- 1 cup no•sugar•added marinara sauce

Instructions:

1. Preheat your oven to 375°F. Lightly grease a baking sheet.

2. Arrange the eggplant slices in a single layer on the prepared baking sheet. Brush the eggplant slices lightly with olive oil on both sides.

3. Bake the eggplant for 12•15 minutes, flipping halfway, until tender and lightly browned.

4. In a medium bowl, mix together the ricotta cheese, Parmesan cheese, beaten egg, chopped basil, and minced garlic. Season with salt and pepper.

5. Spread about 2•3 tablespoons of the ricotta mixture onto the end of each baked eggplant slice. Carefully roll up the eggplant around the filling.

6. Arrange the eggplant rollatini seam•side down in a baking dish. Pour the marinara sauce over the top.

7. Bake the eggplant rollatini for 20•25 minutes, until heated through. Serve the Eggplant Rollatini with Marinara warm.

Tips:
• The Galveston Diet recommends using part•skim ricotta cheese to reduce fat and calories.
• No•sugar•added marinara sauce helps control sugar intake during menopause.
• Eggplant is a nutrient•dense vegetable that provides fiber and antioxidants.

81. Quinoa and Black Bean Stuffed Peppers

Ingredient:

• 4 bell peppers, halved lengthwise and seeds removed
• 1 cup cooked quinoa
• 1 (15 oz) can no•salt•added black beans, rinsed and drained
• 1 cup diced tomatoes
• 1/2 cup crumbled feta cheese
• 2 tablespoons chopped fresh cilantro
• 1 garlic clove, minced
• 1 teaspoon ground cumin
• 1/4 teaspoon chili powder
• Salt and pepper to taste

Instructions:

1. Preheat your oven to 375°F. Place the bell pepper halves in a baking dish and set aside.

2. In a medium bowl, combine the cooked quinoa, black beans, diced tomatoes, feta cheese, chopped cilantro, minced garlic, cumin, and chili powder. Mix well and season with salt and pepper to taste.

3. Spoon the quinoa and black bean mixture evenly into the bell pepper halves, packing it in gently.

4. Cover the baking dish with foil and bake for 25•30 minutes, until the peppers are tender.

5. Remove the foil and bake for an additional 5•10 minutes, until the tops are lightly browned.

6. Serve the Quinoa and Black Bean Stuffed Peppers warm.

Tips:
• The Galveston Diet recommends using no•salt•added canned beans to control sodium intake.
• Quinoa is a nutrient•dense whole grain that provides protein and fiber.
• Feta cheese adds a tangy, creamy element without the need for heavy sauces.
• Spices like cumin and chili powder provide flavor without the use of high•sodium seasonings.

82. Grilled Pork Tenderloin with Apple Chutney

Ingredient:

For the Pork Tenderloin:
• 1 lb pork tenderloin
• 1 tablespoon olive oil
• 1 teaspoon dried thyme
• Salt and pepper to taste

For the Apple Chutney:
• 2 apples, peeled, cored, and diced
• 1 onion, diced
• 2 tablespoons apple cider vinegar
• 1 tablespoon honey
• 1 teaspoon ground cinnamon
• 1/4 teaspoon ground cloves
• Salt and pepper to taste

Instructions:

1. Preheat your grill or grill pan to medium•high heat.

2. Rub the pork tenderloin all over with the olive oil, dried thyme, salt, and pepper.

3. Grill the pork tenderloin for 12•15 minutes per side, or until it reaches an internal temperature of 145°F. Transfer the grilled pork to a cutting board and let it rest for 5 minutes before slicing.

4. While the pork is resting, make the apple chutney. In a small saucepan, combine the diced apples, diced onion, apple cider vinegar, honey, cinnamon, and cloves. Season with salt and pepper.

5. Cook the apple chutney over medium heat, stirring occasionally, for 10•12 minutes, until the apples are softened and the flavors have melded. Slice the grilled pork tenderloin and serve it warm, topped with the apple chutney.

Tips:
• The Galveston Diet encourages the use of lean protein sources like pork tenderloin.
• Grilling the pork adds a nice smoky flavor without the need for heavy sauces or marinades.
• The apple chutney provides a sweet and tangy complement to the savory pork, without the use of high•sugar ingredients.
• This dish is a great source of protein, fiber, and antioxidants.

83. Tomato Basil Mozzarella Salad

Ingredient:

• 2 cups cherry or grape tomatoes, halved
• 8 oz fresh mozzarella cheese, cubed
• 1/4 cup fresh basil leaves, chopped
• 1 tablespoon olive oil
• 1 tablespoon balsamic vinegar
• 1 teaspoon Dijon mustard
• 1 garlic clove, minced
• Salt and pepper to taste

Instructions:

1. In a large bowl, combine the halved tomatoes, cubed mozzarella, and chopped basil leaves.

2. In a small bowl, whisk together the olive oil, balsamic vinegar, Dijon mustard, and minced garlic.

3. Pour the dressing over the tomato, mozzarella, and basil mixture. Gently toss to coat everything evenly.

4. Season the salad with salt and pepper to taste.

5. Serve the Tomato Basil Mozzarella Salad immediately, or chill in the refrigerator for 30 minutes to allow the flavors to meld.

Tips:
• The Galveston Diet encourages the use of healthy fats like those found in olive oil.

• Fresh mozzarella cheese is a low•fat dairy option that fits well within the diet.

• Tomatoes and basil provide antioxidants and anti•inflammatory benefits.

• Balsamic vinegar and Dijon mustard create a flavorful dressing without the need for heavy creams or oils.

This Tomato Basil Mozzarella Salad is a refreshing, nutrient•dense, and easy•to•prepare dish that aligns with the Galveston Diet guidelines during menopause. It makes a great light lunch or side salad.

84. Butternut Squash and Sage Risotto

Ingredient:

• 1 lb butternut squash, peeled, seeded, and cubed
• 2 tablespoons olive oil, divided
• 1 onion, diced
• 2 garlic cloves, minced
• 1 cup arborio rice
• 1/2 cup dry white wine
• 4 cups low•sodium vegetable or chicken broth, heated
• 2 tablespoons chopped fresh sage
• 1/4 cup grated Parmesan cheese
• Salt and pepper to taste

Instructions:

1. Preheat your oven to 400°F. Toss the cubed butternut squash with 1 tablespoon of olive oil and spread it out on a baking sheet. Roast for 20•25 minutes, until tender and lightly browned. Set aside.

2. In a large saucepan, heat the remaining 1 tablespoon of olive oil over medium heat. Add the diced onion and sauté for 3•4 minutes until translucent.

3. Add the minced garlic and arborio rice to the pan. Stir to coat the rice with the oil and cook for 1•2 minutes.

4. Pour in the white wine and stir constantly until the wine is absorbed, about 2 minutes.

5. Add the heated broth to the pan, 1/2 cup at a time, stirring constantly and allowing each addition to be absorbed before adding more. Continue this process until the rice is tender and creamy, about 20•25 minutes total.

6. Stir in the roasted butternut squash and chopped fresh sage. Season with salt and pepper to taste. Remove the risotto from heat and stir in the grated Parmesan cheese. Serve the Butternut Squash and Sage Risotto warm.

Tips:
• The Galveston Diet recommends using low•sodium broth to control sodium intake.
• Arborio rice is a short•grain rice that creates a creamy, risotto•like texture.
• Butternut squash and sage provide a delicious, autumnal flavor profile.
• Parmesan cheese adds a touch of creaminess without the need for heavy cream.

85. Greek Lemon Chicken Soup

Ingredient:

• 1 lb boneless, skinless chicken breasts, cut into bite•sized pieces
• 4 cups low•sodium chicken broth
• 1 cup water
• 2 carrots, peeled and sliced
• 2 celery stalks, sliced
• 1 onion, diced
• 3 garlic cloves, minced
• 1 bay leaf
• 1 teaspoon dried oregano
• 1/4 cup fresh lemon juice
• 2 eggs, beaten
• 2 tablespoons chopped fresh dill
• Salt and pepper to taste

Instructions:

1. In a large pot or Dutch oven, combine the chicken broth, water, carrots, celery, onion, garlic, bay leaf, and dried oregano. Bring to a boil over high heat.

2. Reduce the heat to medium•low and add the chicken pieces. Simmer for 15•20 minutes, or until the chicken is cooked through.

3. Remove the bay leaf. Slowly drizzle the beaten eggs into the simmering soup, stirring constantly, to create egg strands.

4. Stir in the fresh lemon juice and chopped dill. Season with salt and pepper to taste.

5. Serve the Greek Lemon Chicken Soup hot.

Tips:
• The Galveston Diet recommends using low•sodium chicken broth to control sodium intake.
• Chicken is a lean protein source that is suitable for the Galveston Diet.
• Lemon juice and dill add bright, fresh flavors without the need for heavy creams or oils.
• Eggs provide additional protein and create a velvety texture in the soup.

This Greek Lemon Chicken Soup is a comforting, nutrient•dense, and flavorful dish that fits perfectly within the Galveston Diet guidelines during menopause.

86. Stuffed Cabbage Rolls

Ingredient:

• 1 medium head green cabbage
• 1 lb ground turkey or lean ground beef
• 1 cup cooked quinoa
• 1 onion, finely chopped
• 2 garlic cloves, minced
• 1 egg, beaten
• 1 teaspoon dried oregano
• 1/2 teaspoon dried basil
• Salt and pepper to taste
• 1 (15 oz) can no•salt•added diced tomatoes
• 1 cup low•sodium tomato sauce

Instructions:

1. Bring a large pot of water to a boil. Core the cabbage and carefully place it in the boiling water. Cook for 3•5 minutes, until the outer leaves are softened. Remove the cabbage and let cool.

2. Carefully peel off the softened cabbage leaves, keeping them intact. You should have about 12•14 leaves.

3. In a large bowl, combine the ground turkey/beef, cooked quinoa, chopped onion, minced garlic, beaten egg, oregano, basil, salt, and pepper. Mix well.

4. Place about 1/4 cup of the meat mixture onto the center of each cabbage leaf. Fold the sides of the leaf over the filling, then roll up tightly.

5. Arrange the stuffed cabbage rolls seam•side down in a baking dish. Pour the diced tomatoes and tomato sauce over the top.

6. Cover the dish and bake at 375°F for 45•60 minutes, until the cabbage is tender and the filling is cooked through. Serve the Stuffed Cabbage Rolls warm.

Tips:
• The Galveston Diet recommends using lean protein sources like ground turkey or lean beef.
• Quinoa is a whole grain that provides fiber and protein.
• No•salt•added canned tomatoes and low•sodium tomato sauce help control sodium intake.

87. Balsamic Glazed Chicken with Roasted Vegetables

Ingredient:

• 4 boneless, skinless chicken breasts
• 2 tablespoons balsamic vinegar
• 1 tablespoon honey
• 1 teaspoon Dijon mustard
• 1 tablespoon olive oil
• 1 lb Brussels sprouts, trimmed and halved
• 2 cups cubed butternut squash
• 1 red onion, cut into wedges
• 2 garlic cloves, minced
• Salt and pepper to taste
• Chopped fresh parsley for garnish

Instructions:

1. Preheat your oven to 400°F. Line a large baking sheet with parchment paper.

2. In a small bowl, whisk together the balsamic vinegar, honey, and Dijon mustard. Set aside.

3. Place the chicken breasts, Brussels sprouts, butternut squash, and red onion wedges on the prepared baking sheet. Drizzle with the olive oil and season with salt and pepper.

4. Roast the vegetables and chicken for 20 minutes.

5. Remove the baking sheet from the oven and brush the chicken breasts with the balsamic glaze. Return the sheet to the oven and continue roasting for an additional 10•15 minutes, or until the chicken is cooked through and the vegetables are tender.

6. Sprinkle the minced garlic over the roasted vegetables during the last 5 minutes of cooking.

7. Serve the Balsamic Glazed Chicken with the roasted vegetables. Garnish with chopped fresh parsley.

Tips:
• The Galveston Diet encourages the use of lean protein sources like chicken breast.
• Balsamic vinegar and honey create a flavorful glaze without the need for heavy sauces.
• Roasting the vegetables brings out their natural sweetness and nutrients.
• This dish is a complete, balanced meal that fits well within the Galveston Diet guidelines

88. Quinoa and Edamame Salad

Ingredient:

• 1 cup cooked quinoa, cooled
• 1 cup shelled edamame, cooked according to package instructions and cooled
• 1 cup diced cucumber
• 1/2 cup diced red bell pepper
• 1/4 cup chopped green onions
• 2 tablespoons chopped fresh cilantro
• 2 tablespoons rice vinegar
• 1 tablespoon sesame oil
• 1 teaspoon Dijon mustard
• 1 teaspoon honey
• Salt and pepper to taste

Instructions:

1. In a large bowl, combine the cooked and cooled quinoa, edamame, diced cucumber, diced red bell pepper, chopped green onions, and chopped cilantro.

2. In a small bowl, whisk together the rice vinegar, sesame oil, Dijon mustard, and honey. Season with salt and pepper to taste.

3. Pour the dressing over the quinoa and edamame mixture and toss gently to coat everything evenly.

4. Refrigerate the Quinoa and Edamame Salad for at least 30 minutes to allow the flavors to meld.

5. Serve chilled or at room temperature.

Tips:
• The Galveston Diet encourages the use of whole grains like quinoa, which is high in protein and fiber.
• Edamame provides additional plant•based protein and fiber.
• The combination of vegetables, herbs, and a light vinaigrette dressing creates a refreshing and flavorful salad.
• This dish can be served as a main course or a side salad.

The Quinoa and Edamame Salad is a nutritious, easy•to•prepare, and delicious option that fits well within the Galveston Diet guidelines during menopause.

89. Mediterranean Grilled Veggie Wraps

Ingredient:
• 1 zucchini, sliced lengthwise into 1/4•inch thick strips
• 1 red bell pepper, sliced into strips
• 1 yellow squash, sliced lengthwise into 1/4•inch thick strips
• 1 eggplant, sliced lengthwise into 1/4•inch thick strips
• 2 tablespoons olive oil
• 1 teaspoon dried oregano
• Salt and pepper to taste
• 4 whole wheat tortillas or wraps
• 1/2 cup crumbled feta cheese
• 1/4 cup pitted kalamata olives, sliced
• 2 tablespoons chopped fresh basil

Instructions:
1. Preheat your grill or grill pan to medium•high heat.

2. In a large bowl, toss the sliced zucchini, bell pepper, yellow squash, and eggplant with the olive oil, dried oregano, salt, and pepper.

3. Grill the vegetables for 3•4 minutes per side, until they are tender and have grill marks.

4. Remove the grilled vegetables from the grill and let them cool slightly.

5. Lay the whole wheat tortillas or wraps on a flat surface. Divide the grilled vegetables evenly among the tortillas, placing them in the center.

6. Top the grilled veggies with crumbled feta cheese, sliced kalamata olives, and chopped fresh basil.

7. Fold the bottom of the tortilla up over the filling, then fold in the sides and continue rolling tightly to create a wrap. Serve the Mediterranean Grilled Veggie Wraps immediately.

Tips:
• The Galveston Diet encourages the use of whole grains, like whole wheat tortillas, to provide fiber and complex carbohydrates.
• Grilling the vegetables adds a delicious smoky flavor without the need for heavy sauces or dressings.
• Feta cheese, olives, and fresh basil provide Mediterranean flavors that complement the grilled veggies

90. Tuna Stuffed Bell Peppers

Ingredient:

• 4 bell peppers (any color)
• 1 (5 oz) can tuna, drained
• 1/4 cup cooked rice
• 2 tbsp mayonnaise
• 1 tbsp finely chopped onion
• 1 tsp Dijon mustard
• Salt and pepper to taste
• Shredded cheese (optional)

Instructions:

1. Preheat oven to 375°F.

2. Cut the tops off the bell peppers and remove the seeds and membranes. Place the peppers in a baking dish.

3. In a medium bowl, mix together the tuna, cooked rice, mayonnaise, onion, Dijon mustard, salt, and pepper until well combined.

4. Spoon the tuna mixture evenly into the hollowed out bell peppers.

5. If desired, top the stuffed peppers with shredded cheese.

6. Bake for 20•25 minutes, until the peppers are tender and the filling is heated through.

7. Serve hot. Enjoy!

The tuna and rice filling provides a tasty and protein•packed stuffing for the bell peppers. This makes a great light main dish or appetizer. Feel free to adjust the seasonings to your taste.

91. Spicy Thai Peanut Chicken Stir•Fry

Ingredient:

• 1 lb boneless, skinless chicken breasts, cut into 1•inch pieces
• 2 tbsp coconut oil
• 1 red bell pepper, sliced
• 1 cup broccoli florets
• 1 cup snow peas
• 3 cloves garlic, minced
• 1 tbsp grated fresh ginger
• 2 tbsp low•sodium soy sauce
• 2 tbsp natural peanut butter
• 1 tbsp rice vinegar
• 1 tsp red pepper flakes (or to taste)
• 1/4 cup chopped fresh cilantro
• 2 tbsp chopped roasted peanuts (optional)

Instructions:

1. Heat the coconut oil in a large skillet or wok over medium•high heat.

2. Add the chicken and stir•fry for 5•7 minutes until cooked through. Remove the chicken from the pan and set aside.

3. Add the bell pepper, broccoli, and snow peas to the pan. Stir•fry for 3•4 minutes until the vegetables are crisp•tender.

4. Add the garlic and ginger and cook for 1 minute, stirring constantly.

5. In a small bowl, whisk together the soy sauce, peanut butter, rice vinegar, and red pepper flakes.

6. Add the cooked chicken back to the pan and pour the peanut sauce over the top. Toss everything together until well coated.

7. Remove from heat and stir in the chopped cilantro.

8. Serve immediately, garnished with chopped roasted peanuts if desired.

This stir•fry is packed with protein, vegetables, and a flavorful peanut sauce. It's a great option for the Galveston Diet and menopause as it's low in carbs, high in fiber, and contains healthy fats from the peanut butter and coconut oil.

92. Roasted Cauliflower Steaks with Tahini Sauce

Ingredient:

For the Cauliflower Steaks:
• 1 large head of cauliflower, cut into 1•inch thick slices
• 2 tbsp olive oil
• Salt and pepper to taste

For the Tahini Sauce:
• 1/4 cup tahini
• 2 tbsp lemon juice
• 2 tbsp water
• 1 garlic clove, minced
• 1/4 tsp ground cumin
• Salt and pepper to taste

Instructions:

1. Preheat your oven to 400°F.

2. Lay the cauliflower slices on a large baking sheet. Brush both sides with olive oil and season with salt and pepper.

3. Roast the cauliflower for 20•25 minutes, flipping halfway, until tender and lightly browned.

4. While the cauliflower is roasting, make the tahini sauce. In a small bowl, whisk together the tahini, lemon juice, water, garlic, cumin, salt, and pepper until smooth and creamy.

5. Serve the roasted cauliflower steaks warm, drizzled with the tahini sauce. Garnish with chopped parsley or cilantro if desired.

This dish is a great option for the Galveston Diet and menopause for a few reasons:

• Cauliflower is a low•carb, high•fiber vegetable that is rich in nutrients like vitamin C, vitamin K, and folate.
• Tahini is a good source of healthy fats, protein, and minerals like calcium and magnesium.
• The dish is gluten•free, dairy•free, and plant•based, making it suitable for various dietary needs.
• The combination of roasted cauliflower and creamy tahini sauce provides a satisfying and flavorful meal.

93. Beet and Quinoa Salad with Goat Cheese

Ingredient:

• 1 cup cooked quinoa, cooled
• 3 medium beets, roasted and diced
• 1/2 cup crumbled goat cheese
• 1/4 cup chopped walnuts
• 2 tbsp chopped fresh parsley
• 2 tbsp olive oil
• 1 tbsp balsamic vinegar
• 1 tsp Dijon mustard
• Salt and pepper to taste

Instructions:

1. Preheat oven to 400°F. Wrap the beets in foil and roast for 45•60 minutes, until tender when pierced with a fork. Allow to cool, then peel and dice the beets.

2. In a large bowl, combine the cooked quinoa, diced beets, crumbled goat cheese, chopped walnuts, and parsley.

3. In a small bowl, whisk together the olive oil, balsamic vinegar, and Dijon mustard. Season with salt and pepper.

4. Pour the dressing over the quinoa and beet mixture and toss gently to coat.

5. Serve chilled or at room temperature. Enjoy!

This Beet and Quinoa Salad is a great option for a healthy, nutrient•dense meal. The combination of earthy beets, protein•rich quinoa, creamy goat cheese, and crunchy walnuts makes for a satisfying and flavorful salad.

Some of the key benefits of this dish:

• Beets are a great source of fiber, folate, manganese, and antioxidants.
• Quinoa is a gluten•free grain that is high in protein, fiber, and minerals.
• Goat cheese provides calcium and probiotics.
• Walnuts add healthy fats and crunch.

This salad can be enjoyed as a main dish or side. It's a great option for the Galveston Diet and menopause due to the nutrient•dense ingredients.

94. Garlic Shrimp with Zucchini Noodles

Ingredient:

- 1 lb large shrimp, peeled and deveined
- 2 tbsp olive oil
- 4 cloves garlic, minced
- 1 tsp red pepper flakes (optional)
- 1/4 cup dry white wine or low•sodium chicken broth
- 2 medium zucchini, spiralized or julienned into noodles
- 2 tbsp chopped fresh parsley
- Salt and pepper to taste

Instructions:

1. In a large skillet, heat the olive oil over medium•high heat. Add the shrimp, garlic, and red pepper flakes (if using). Cook for 2•3 minutes, stirring frequently, until the shrimp start to turn pink.

2. Pour in the white wine or broth and let it simmer for 1•2 minutes, scraping up any browned bits from the bottom of the pan.

3. Add the zucchini noodles to the pan and toss everything together. Cook for 2•3 minutes, just until the zucchini is tender but still has some bite.

4. Remove from heat and stir in the chopped parsley. Season with salt and pepper to taste.

5. Serve the garlic shrimp and zucchini noodles immediately, while hot.

This dish is a great option for the Galveston Diet and menopause for a few reasons:

- Shrimp is a lean protein that is low in calories and high in nutrients like selenium and vitamin B12.
- Zucchini noodles are a low•carb, high•fiber alternative to traditional pasta.
- The dish is gluten•free, dairy•free, and keto•friendly.
- The garlic, olive oil, and parsley provide anti•inflammatory benefits.

The combination of tender shrimp, flavorful garlic, and nutrient•dense zucchini noodles makes for a satisfying and healthy meal. Enjoy!

95. Greek Stuffed Chicken Breast

Ingredient:

• 4 boneless, skinless chicken breasts
• 1/2 cup crumbled feta cheese
• 1/4 cup chopped sun•dried tomatoes
• 2 tbsp chopped fresh spinach
• 1 tbsp chopped fresh oregano
• 1 tsp minced garlic
• Salt and pepper to taste
• 1 tbsp olive oil

For the Sauce:
• 1/2 cup plain Greek yogurt
• 1 tbsp lemon juice
• 1 tsp minced garlic
• Salt and pepper to taste

Instructions:

1. Preheat your oven to 400°F.

2. In a medium bowl, mix together the feta cheese, sun•dried tomatoes, spinach, oregano, and garlic. Season with salt and pepper.

3. Slice each chicken breast horizontally to create a pocket. Stuff each pocket with the feta mixture, dividing it evenly.

4. Heat the olive oil in a large oven•safe skillet over medium•high heat. Add the stuffed chicken breasts and sear for 2•3 minutes per side to get a nice golden•brown crust.

5. Transfer the skillet to the preheated oven and bake for 15•20 minutes, until the chicken is cooked through and the internal temperature reaches 165°F.

6. While the chicken is baking, make the sauce. In a small bowl, whisk together the Greek yogurt, lemon juice, garlic, salt, and pepper. Serve the Greek stuffed chicken breasts warm, drizzled with the yogurt sauce. Enjoy!

This dish is a great option for the Galveston Diet and menopause for a few reasons:

• Chicken is a lean protein that is low in calories and high in nutrients.
• Feta cheese provides calcium and probiotics.
• Sun•dried tomatoes and spinach are rich in antioxidants and fiber.
• The yogurt sauce adds a creamy, tangy element to the dish.

96. Lentil and Vegetable Soup

Ingredient:

• 1 tbsp olive oil
• 1 onion, diced
• 3 cloves garlic, minced
• 2 carrots, peeled and diced
• 2 celery stalks, diced
• 1 cup green or brown lentils, rinsed
• 6 cups low•sodium vegetable or chicken broth
• 1 (14.5 oz) can diced tomatoes
• 2 cups chopped kale or spinach
• 1 tsp dried thyme
• 1 tsp dried oregano
• Salt and pepper to taste

Instructions:

1. In a large pot or Dutch oven, heat the olive oil over medium heat. Add the onion and sauté for 3•4 minutes until translucent.

2. Add the garlic, carrots, and celery. Cook for another 2•3 minutes, stirring frequently.

3. Stir in the lentils, broth, diced tomatoes, kale/spinach, thyme, and oregano. Season with salt and pepper.

4. Bring the soup to a boil, then reduce heat and let it simmer for 20•25 minutes, or until the lentils are tender.

5. Taste and adjust seasoning as needed. Serve the lentil and vegetable soup hot, garnished with extra chopped kale or parsley if desired.

This soup is an excellent choice for the Galveston Diet and menopause for several reasons:

• Lentils are a great source of plant•based protein, fiber, and complex carbs.
• Vegetables like carrots, celery, and kale/spinach provide a variety of vitamins, minerals, and antioxidants.
• The soup is low in calories and fat, but high in nutrients.
• The herbs and spices add flavor without the need for excessive sodium.

97. Ratatouille Stuffed Zucchini

Ingredient:

- 4 medium zucchini, halved lengthwise
- 1 tbsp olive oil
- 1 onion, diced
- 2 cloves garlic, minced
- 1 eggplant, diced

- 1 red bell pepper, diced
- 1 can (14.5 oz) diced tomatoes
- 2 tbsp chopped fresh basil
- 1 tsp dried oregano
- Salt and pepper to taste
- 1/2 cup crumbled feta cheese (optional)

Instructions:

1. Preheat your oven to 400°F.

2. Scoop out the flesh from the zucchini halves, leaving about 1/4 inch of the zucchini shell. Chop the scooped•out zucchini flesh.

3. In a large skillet, heat the olive oil over medium heat. Add the onion and sauté for 3•4 minutes until translucent.

4. Add the garlic, chopped zucchini flesh, eggplant, and bell pepper. Cook for 5•7 minutes, stirring occasionally, until the vegetables are tender.

5. Stir in the diced tomatoes, basil, oregano, salt, and pepper. Simmer for 5•10 minutes, allowing the flavors to meld.

6. Arrange the zucchini shells in a baking dish. Spoon the ratatouille mixture evenly into the zucchini shells. If desired, sprinkle the tops with crumbled feta cheese.

8. Bake for 20•25 minutes, until the zucchini is tender and the filling is hot. Serve the ratatouille stuffed zucchini warm.

This dish is a great option for the Galveston Diet and menopause for several reasons:

- Zucchini is a low•carb, high•fiber vegetable that is rich in vitamins and minerals.

- The ratatouille filling is packed with antioxidant•rich vegetables like eggplant, bell pepper, and tomatoes.

- The dish is gluten•free, dairy•free (without the optional feta), and plant•based.

- The combination of vegetables and herbs provides anti•inflammatory benefits.

98. Baked Stuffed Mushrooms with Spinach and Cheese

Ingredient:

- 1/4 cup grated Parmesan cheese
- 2 oz cream cheese, softened
- 1/4 tsp dried thyme
- Salt and pepper to taste

- 12 large mushrooms, stems removed and finely chopped
- 1 tbsp olive oil
- 1/2 cup chopped onion
- 2 cloves garlic, minced
- 1 cup fresh spinach, chopped

Instructions:

1. Preheat your oven to 375°F.

2. In a skillet, heat the olive oil over medium heat. Add the chopped mushroom stems, onion, and garlic. Sauté for 3•4 minutes until the vegetables are softened.

3. Add the chopped spinach and continue cooking for 1•2 minutes until the spinach is wilted.

4. Remove the skillet from heat and stir in the Parmesan cheese, cream cheese, and dried thyme. Season with salt and pepper.

5. Stuff the mushroom caps evenly with the spinach and cheese mixture.

6. Arrange the stuffed mushrooms on a baking sheet lined with parchment paper.

7. Bake for 12•15 minutes, until the mushrooms are tender and the filling is hot and bubbly. Serve the baked stuffed mushrooms warm.

This dish is a great option for the Galveston Diet and menopause for several reasons:

- Mushrooms are a low•carb, nutrient•dense vegetable that provides antioxidants and B vitamins.
- Spinach is a leafy green that is rich in vitamins, minerals, and fiber.
- Parmesan cheese and cream cheese provide calcium and healthy fats.
- The dish is gluten•free and can be easily adapted to be dairy•free by using a non•dairy cream cheese alternative.

The combination of the savory mushroom caps, creamy spinach and cheese filling, and the baked texture makes these stuffed mushrooms a delicious and satisfying appetizer or side dish. Enjoy this healthy and flavorful recipe!

99. Quinoa and Chickpea Tabbouleh

Ingredient:

- 1 cup cooked quinoa, cooled
- 1 (15 oz) can chickpeas, rinsed and drained
- 1 cup diced cucumber
- 1 cup diced tomatoes
- 1/2 cup chopped fresh parsley
- 1/4 cup chopped fresh mint
- 2 tbsp lemon juice
- 1 tbsp olive oil
- 1 clove garlic, minced
- 1/4 tsp ground cumin
- Salt and pepper to taste

Instructions:

1. In a large bowl, combine the cooked quinoa, chickpeas, cucumber, tomatoes, parsley, and mint.

2. In a small bowl, whisk together the lemon juice, olive oil, garlic, and cumin. Season with salt and pepper.

3. Pour the dressing over the quinoa and chickpea mixture and toss gently to coat.

4. Refrigerate the tabbouleh for at least 30 minutes to allow the flavors to meld.

5. Serve chilled or at room temperature.

This Quinoa and Chickpea Tabbouleh is an excellent choice for the Galveston Diet and menopause for several reasons:

- Quinoa is a gluten•free, high•protein grain that provides complex carbs and fiber.
- Chickpeas are a good source of plant•based protein, fiber, and minerals.
- Vegetables like cucumber and tomatoes are rich in vitamins, minerals, and antioxidants.
- Fresh herbs like parsley and mint add flavor and anti•inflammatory benefits.
- The lemon juice, olive oil, and garlic provide a light, flavorful dressing.

The combination of nutrient•dense ingredients makes this tabbouleh a satisfying and healthy meal or side dish. It's perfect for the Galveston Diet and can help support overall health during menopause.

100. Grilled Chicken and Vegetable Skewers with Lemon Herb Marinade

Ingredient:

• 1/4 cup olive oil
• 2 tbsp lemon juice
• 2 tbsp chopped fresh parsley
• 1 tbsp chopped fresh oregano
• 2 cloves garlic, minced
• 1 tsp Dijon mustard
• Salt and pepper to taste

Skewer Ingredients:

• 1 lb boneless, skinless chicken breasts, cut into 1•inch cubes
• 1 zucchini, cut into 1•inch pieces
• 1 red bell pepper, cut into 1•inch pieces
• 1 yellow onion, cut into 1•inch pieces
• 8•10 cherry tomatoes

Instructions:

1. In a medium bowl, whisk together all the marinade ingredients. Add the chicken cubes and toss to coat. Cover and refrigerate for 30 minutes to 1 hour.

2. Preheat your grill or grill pan to medium•high heat.

3. Thread the marinated chicken, zucchini, bell pepper, onion, and cherry tomatoes onto metal or wooden skewers.

4. Grill the skewers for 12•15 minutes, turning occasionally, until the chicken is cooked through and the vegetables are tender.

5. Serve the grilled chicken and vegetable skewers immediately, with any remaining marinade drizzled over the top.

This dish is an excellent choice for the Galveston Diet and menopause for several reasons:

• Chicken is a lean protein that is low in calories and high in nutrients.
• Vegetables like zucchini, bell pepper, and onion provide fiber, vitamins, and antioxidants.
• The lemon, herbs, and Dijon mustard in the marinade add flavor without the need for excessive sodium.
• The dish is gluten•free, dairy•free, and keto•friendly.

101. Mediterranean Orzo Salad

Ingredient:

- 1 cup uncooked orzo pasta
- 1 cup cherry tomatoes, halved
- 1 cucumber, diced
- 1/2 cup crumbled feta cheese
- 1/4 cup kalamata olives, sliced
- 1/4 cup chopped fresh parsley
- 2 tbsp chopped fresh basil
- 2 tbsp olive oil
- 2 tbsp lemon juice
- 1 tsp Dijon mustard
- 1 clove garlic, minced
- Salt and pepper to taste

Instructions:

1. Cook the orzo according to package instructions. Drain and rinse with cold water to cool completely.

2. In a large bowl, combine the cooked and cooled orzo, cherry tomatoes, cucumber, feta cheese, olives, parsley, and basil.

3. In a small bowl, whisk together the olive oil, lemon juice, Dijon mustard, and garlic. Season with salt and pepper.

4. Pour the dressing over the orzo salad and toss gently to coat.

5. Refrigerate the salad for at least 30 minutes to allow the flavors to meld.

6. Serve chilled or at room temperature.

This Mediterranean Orzo Salad is an excellent choice for the Galveston Diet and menopause for several reasons:

- Orzo is a small, rice•shaped pasta that provides complex carbs and fiber.
- Vegetables like tomatoes, cucumber, and olives are rich in antioxidants and vitamins.
- Feta cheese is a good source of calcium and probiotics.
- Fresh herbs like parsley and basil add flavor and anti•inflammatory benefits.
- The olive oil and lemon juice dressing is light and flavorful without the need for excessive sodium.

The combination of Mediterranean•inspired ingredients makes this salad a refreshing and nutritious meal or side dish. It's perfect for the Galveston Diet and can help support overall health during menopause.

102. Sweet Potato and Black Bean Buddha Bowl

Ingredient:

• 2 medium sweet potatoes, peeled and cubed
• 1 tbsp olive oil
• 1 (15 oz) can black beans, rinsed and drained
• 1 cup cooked quinoa
• 1 cup shredded red cabbage
• 1 avocado, sliced
• 2 tbsp toasted pumpkin seeds
• 2 tbsp chopped fresh cilantro

For the Dressing:
• 2 tbsp tahini
• 2 tbsp lemon juice
• 1 tbsp water
• 1 tsp honey
• 1 clove garlic, minced
• Salt and pepper to taste

Instructions:

1. Preheat your oven to 400°F. Toss the cubed sweet potatoes with the olive oil and spread them on a baking sheet. Roast for 20•25 minutes, until tender and lightly browned.

2. In a large bowl, combine the roasted sweet potatoes, black beans, cooked quinoa, shredded cabbage, avocado slices, pumpkin seeds, and chopped cilantro.

3. In a small bowl, whisk together all the dressing ingredients until smooth and creamy. Season with salt and pepper.

4. Drizzle the tahini dressing over the Buddha bowl and gently toss to coat. Serve the Sweet Potato and Black Bean Buddha Bowl immediately.

This dish is an excellent choice for the Galveston Diet and menopause for several reasons:

• Sweet potatoes are a nutrient•dense carbohydrate that provides fiber, vitamins, and antioxidants.
• Black beans are a good source of plant•based protein, fiber, and complex carbs.
• Quinoa is a gluten•free, high•protein grain that adds texture and nutrients.
• Vegetables like cabbage and avocado provide additional fiber, vitamins, and healthy fats.
• The tahini•based dressing is a good source of calcium and healthy fats.

The combination of these wholesome, plant•based ingredients makes this Buddha bowl a satisfying and nutritious meal. It's perfect for the Galveston Diet and can help support overall health during menopause.

103. Shrimp and Avocado Salad

Ingredient:

• 1 lb cooked shrimp, peeled and deveined
• 2 avocados, diced
• 1 cup cherry tomatoes, halved
• 1/2 red onion, thinly sliced
• 1/4 cup chopped fresh cilantro
• 2 tbsp olive oil
• 2 tbsp lime juice
• 1 tsp Dijon mustard
• Salt and pepper to taste

Instructions:

1. In a large bowl, gently combine the cooked shrimp, diced avocados, cherry tomatoes, red onion, and chopped cilantro.

2. In a small bowl, whisk together the olive oil, lime juice, and Dijon mustard. Season with salt and pepper.

3. Pour the dressing over the shrimp and avocado mixture and toss gently to coat.

4. Refrigerate the salad for at least 30 minutes to allow the flavors to meld.

5. Serve chilled or at room temperature.

This Shrimp and Avocado Salad is a great option for the Galveston Diet and menopause for several reasons:

• Shrimp is a lean protein that is low in calories and high in nutrients like selenium and vitamin B12.
• Avocados are a good source of healthy monounsaturated fats, fiber, and antioxidants.
• Cherry tomatoes and red onion provide additional vitamins, minerals, and phytochemicals.
• The fresh cilantro adds an anti•inflammatory boost.
• The simple dressing of olive oil, lime juice, and Dijon mustard is light and flavorful.

The combination of protein•rich shrimp, creamy avocado, and fresh vegetables makes this salad a satisfying and nutritious meal. It's perfect for the Galveston Diet and can help support overall health during menopause.

104. Caprese Quinoa Salad

Ingredient:

• 1 cup cooked quinoa, cooled
• 1 cup cherry tomatoes, halved
• 1 cup fresh mozzarella cheese, cubed
• 1/4 cup fresh basil leaves, chopped
• 2 tbsp balsamic glaze
• 1 tbsp olive oil
• 1 tbsp lemon juice
• Salt and pepper to taste

Instructions:

1. In a large bowl, combine the cooked and cooled quinoa, cherry tomatoes, mozzarella cheese, and chopped basil.

2. In a small bowl, whisk together the balsamic glaze, olive oil, and lemon juice. Season with salt and pepper.

3. Pour the dressing over the quinoa salad and toss gently to coat.

4. Refrigerate the salad for at least 30 minutes to allow the flavors to meld.

5. Serve chilled or at room temperature.

This Caprese Quinoa Salad is a great option for the Galveston Diet and menopause for several reasons:

• Quinoa is a gluten•free, high•protein grain that provides complex carbs and fiber.
• Cherry tomatoes are a good source of vitamins C and K, as well as the antioxidant lycopene.
• Fresh mozzarella cheese is a source of calcium and probiotics.
• Basil is an anti•inflammatory herb that adds flavor and nutrients.
• The balsamic glaze and lemon juice provide a tangy, low•calorie dressing.

The combination of nutrient•dense ingredients makes this salad a satisfying and healthy meal or side dish. It's perfect for the Galveston Diet and can help support overall health during menopause.

105. Baked Cod with Mediterranean Salsa

Ingredient:

For the Salsa:
• 1 cup diced tomatoes
• 1/2 cup diced cucumber
• 1/4 cup diced red onion
• 2 tbsp chopped fresh parsley
• 1 tbsp chopped fresh basil
• 1 tbsp olive oil
• 1 tbsp lemon juice

• 1 clove garlic, minced
• Salt and pepper to taste

For the Cod:
• 4 (6 oz) cod fillets
• 1 tbsp olive oil
• Salt and pepper to taste

Instructions:

1. Preheat your oven to 400°F.

2. In a medium bowl, combine all the salsa ingredients. Stir well and set aside.

3. Pat the cod fillets dry and place them on a baking sheet lined with parchment paper. Brush the cod with the olive oil and season with salt and pepper.

4. Bake the cod for 12•15 minutes, or until it flakes easily with a fork.

5. Serve the baked cod warm, topped with the Mediterranean salsa.

This Baked Cod with Mediterranean Salsa is an excellent choice for the Galveston Diet and menopause for several reasons:

• Cod is a lean, protein•rich fish that is low in calories and high in nutrients like vitamin B12 and selenium.

• The Mediterranean•inspired salsa is packed with fresh vegetables, herbs, and healthy fats from the olive oil.

• The dish is gluten•free, dairy•free, and keto•friendly. The combination of the baked cod and the vibrant salsa provides a flavorful and nutritious meal.

The fresh, bright flavors of the salsa complement the mild, flaky cod perfectly. This dish is a great way to incorporate heart•healthy fish and anti•inflammatory ingredients into your Galveston Diet and menopause•friendly meal plan.

106. Curried Lentil Soup

Ingredient:

- 1 tbsp olive oil
- 1 onion, diced
- 3 cloves garlic, minced
- 1 tbsp grated fresh ginger
- 2 tsp curry powder
- 1 tsp ground cumin
- 1/4 tsp cayenne pepper (optional)
- 1 cup dried red lentils, rinsed
- 4 cups low•sodium vegetable or chicken broth
- 1 (14.5 oz) can diced tomatoes
- 1 cup chopped spinach or kale
- 1 cup unsweetened coconut milk
- Salt and pepper to taste
- Chopped cilantro for garnish (optional)

Instructions:

1. In a large pot or Dutch oven, heat the olive oil over medium heat. Add the onion and sauté for 3•4 minutes until translucent.

2. Add the garlic, ginger, curry powder, cumin, and cayenne (if using). Cook for 1 minute, stirring constantly, until fragrant.

3. Stir in the lentils, broth, and diced tomatoes. Bring the soup to a boil, then reduce heat and let it simmer for 15•20 minutes, until the lentils are tender.

4. Add the chopped spinach or kale and the coconut milk. Simmer for 5 more minutes, until the greens are wilted. Season the soup with salt and pepper to taste. Serve the Curried Lentil Soup hot, garnished with chopped cilantro if desired.

This Curried Lentil Soup is an excellent choice for the Galveston Diet and menopause for several reasons:

- Lentils are a great source of plant•based protein, fiber, and complex carbs.
- Spinach and kale are nutrient•dense leafy greens that provide vitamins, minerals, and antioxidants.
- Coconut milk adds creaminess and healthy fats.
- The curry powder, ginger, and cayenne provide anti•inflammatory benefits.
- The soup is low in calories and high in fiber, making it a filling and satisfying meal.

107. Grilled Vegetable Platter with Hummus

Ingredient:

Vegetables:
• 1 zucchini, sliced into 1/2•inch thick rounds
• 1 yellow squash, sliced into 1/2•inch thick rounds
• 1 red bell pepper, cut into 1•inch pieces
• 1 eggplant, cut into 1/2•inch thick slices
• 1 red onion, cut into 1/2•inch thick slices
• 2 tbsp olive oil
• Salt and pepper to taste

Hummus:
• 1 (15 oz) can chickpeas, rinsed and drained
• 2 tbsp tahini
• 2 tbsp lemon juice
• 1 clove garlic, minced
• 2 tbsp olive oil
• 2 tbsp water
• Salt and pepper to taste

Instructions:

1. Preheat your grill or grill pan to medium•high heat.

2. In a large bowl, toss the sliced vegetables with the 2 tbsp of olive oil. Season with salt and pepper.

3. Grill the vegetables for 3•5 minutes per side, until tender and lightly charred.

4. While the vegetables are grilling, make the hummus. In a food processor, combine the chickpeas, tahini, lemon juice, garlic, 2 tbsp olive oil, and water. Blend until smooth. Season with salt and pepper.

5. Arrange the grilled vegetables on a platter. Serve the homemade hummus alongside the vegetables for dipping.

This Grilled Vegetable Platter with Hummus is an excellent choice for the Galveston Diet and menopause for several reasons:

• The vegetables, such as zucchini, squash, bell pepper, eggplant, and onion, are low in carbs and high in fiber, vitamins, and antioxidants.
• Chickpeas, the main ingredient in the hummus, provide plant•based protein and fiber.
• Tahini, a sesame seed paste, is a good source of calcium and healthy fats.
• The dish is gluten•free, dairy•free, and vegan, making it suitable for various dietary needs.
• The combination of grilled vegetables and nutrient•dense hummus creates a satisfying and nourishing meal or snack

108. Quinoa and Kale Stuffed Bell Peppers

Ingredient:

• 4 bell peppers, halved and seeded
• 1 cup cooked quinoa
• 1 cup chopped kale
• 1/2 cup diced tomatoes
• 1/4 cup crumbled feta cheese
• 2 tbsp chopped fresh basil
• 1 tbsp olive oil
• 1 clove garlic, minced
• Salt and pepper to taste

Instructions:

1. Preheat your oven to 375°F.

2. In a large bowl, combine the cooked quinoa, chopped kale, diced tomatoes, feta cheese, and chopped basil.

3. In a small skillet, heat the olive oil over medium heat. Add the minced garlic and cook for 1 minute, until fragrant.

4. Pour the garlic•infused olive oil into the quinoa and kale mixture. Stir to combine. Season with salt and pepper.

5. Arrange the bell pepper halves in a baking dish. Spoon the quinoa and kale filling evenly into the pepper halves. Bake for 20•25 minutes, until the peppers are tender and the filling is hot. Serve the Quinoa and Kale Stuffed Bell Peppers warm.

This dish is an excellent choice for the Galveston Diet and menopause for several reasons:

• Bell peppers are a low•carb, nutrient•dense vegetable that provides vitamins, minerals, and antioxidants.
• Quinoa is a gluten•free, high•protein grain that adds fiber and complex carbs.
• Kale is a leafy green that is rich in vitamins, minerals, and anti•inflammatory compounds.
• Feta cheese provides calcium and probiotics.
• The dish is low in calories and high in nutrients, making it a satisfying and healthy meal.

The combination of the flavorful quinoa and kale filling and the roasted bell pepper creates a delicious and nutritious dish that is perfect for the Galveston Diet and menopause. Enjoy this Quinoa and Kale Stuffed Bell Peppers recipe!

109. Lemon Garlic Chicken with Asparagus

Ingredient:

• 4 boneless, skinless chicken breasts
• 2 tbsp olive oil
• 3 cloves garlic, minced
• 2 tbsp lemon juice
• 1 tsp lemon zest
• 1 tsp dried oregano
• Salt and pepper to taste
• 1 lb asparagus, trimmed

Instructions:

1. Preheat your oven to 400°F.

2. In a small bowl, combine the olive oil, minced garlic, lemon juice, lemon zest, and dried oregano. Season with salt and pepper.

3. Place the chicken breasts in a baking dish and pour the lemon•garlic mixture over the top, making sure to coat the chicken evenly.

4. Arrange the trimmed asparagus around the chicken in the baking dish.

5. Bake for 20•25 minutes, or until the chicken is cooked through and the asparagus is tender.

6. Serve the Lemon Garlic Chicken immediately, with the asparagus and any pan juices spooned over the top.

This dish is an excellent choice for the Galveston Diet and menopause for several reasons:

• Chicken is a lean protein that is low in calories and high in nutrients like vitamin B6 and niacin.
• Asparagus is a low•carb, fiber•rich vegetable that provides vitamins, minerals, and antioxidants.
• The lemon, garlic, and oregano add flavor without the need for excessive sodium.
• The dish is gluten•free, dairy•free, and keto•friendly.

The bright, lemony flavors and the tender chicken and asparagus make this a delicious and nutritious meal. It's a great option for the Galveston Diet and can help support overall health during menopause.

110. Eggplant and Chickpea Curry

Ingredient:

- 1 medium eggplant, cut into 1•inch cubes
- 1 tbsp olive oil
- 1 onion, diced
- 3 cloves garlic, minced
- 1 tbsp grated fresh ginger
- 2 tsp curry powder
- 1 tsp ground cumin
- 1/4 tsp cayenne pepper (optional)
- 1 (15 oz) can chickpeas, rinsed and drained
- 1 (14.5 oz) can diced tomatoes
- 1 cup low•sodium vegetable or chicken broth
- 1 cup full•fat coconut milk
- Salt and pepper to taste
- Chopped cilantro for garnish (optional)

Instructions:

1. In a large skillet or Dutch oven, heat the olive oil over medium heat. Add the cubed eggplant and sauté for 5•7 minutes, until lightly browned.

2. Add the diced onion and cook for 3•4 minutes, until translucent.

3. Stir in the minced garlic, grated ginger, curry powder, cumin, and cayenne (if using). Cook for 1 minute, until fragrant.

4. Add the chickpeas, diced tomatoes, vegetable/chicken broth, and coconut milk. Bring the mixture to a simmer.

5. Reduce heat to low and let the curry simmer for 15•20 minutes, stirring occasionally, until the eggplant is very tender.

6. Season the curry with salt and pepper to taste. Serve the Eggplant and Chickpea Curry hot, garnished with chopped cilantro if desired. Enjoy with cauliflower rice or naan bread.

This curry dish is an excellent choice for the Galveston Diet and menopause for several reasons:

- Eggplant is a low•carb, fiber•rich vegetable that provides antioxidants.
- Chickpeas are a good source of plant•based protein, fiber, and complex carbs.
- Coconut milk adds creaminess and healthy fats.
- The spices like curry powder, cumin, and ginger provide anti•inflammatory benefits.
- The dish is gluten•free, dairy•free, and vegan, making it suitable for various dietary needs.

The combination of the tender eggplant, protein•packed chickpeas, and aromatic curry flavors makes this a nourishing and satisfying meal. Enjoy this Eggplant and Chickpea Curry as part of your Galveston Diet and menopause•friendly meal plan.

111. Spinach and Feta Stuffed Portobello Mushrooms

Ingredient:

• 4 large portobello mushroom caps, stems removed and chopped
• 2 tbsp olive oil, divided
• 1 shallot, minced
• 2 cloves garlic, minced
• 2 cups fresh spinach, chopped
• 1/2 cup crumbled feta cheese
• 2 tbsp grated Parmesan cheese
• 1 tbsp lemon juice
• Salt and pepper to taste

Instructions:

1. Preheat your oven to 400°F.

2. Brush the portobello mushroom caps with 1 tbsp of the olive oil and place them cap·side down on a baking sheet. Bake for 10 minutes.

3. In a skillet, heat the remaining 1 tbsp of olive oil over medium heat. Add the chopped mushroom stems, shallot, and garlic. Sauté for 2·3 minutes until fragrant.

4. Add the chopped spinach to the skillet and cook for 2·3 minutes, until the spinach is wilted.

5. Remove the skillet from heat and stir in the crumbled feta, Parmesan, and lemon juice. Season with salt and pepper.

6. Flip the baked portobello caps over so they are cap·side up. Spoon the spinach and feta mixture evenly into the mushroom caps.

7. Return the stuffed mushrooms to the oven and bake for an additional 10·12 minutes, until the mushrooms are tender and the filling is hot. Serve the Spinach and Feta Stuffed Portobello Mushrooms warm.

The combination of the savory mushroom caps, creamy spinach and feta filling, and the baked texture makes these stuffed mushrooms a delicious and satisfying meal or appetizer. Enjoy this healthy and flavorful recipe!

112. Zucchini Noodles with Tomato Basil Sauce

Ingredient:

• 3 medium zucchini, spiralized or julienned into noodles
• 2 tbsp olive oil
• 3 cloves garlic, minced
• 1 (14.5 oz) can diced tomatoes
• 1/4 cup fresh basil leaves, chopped
• 2 tbsp tomato paste
• 1 tsp dried oregano
• Salt and pepper to taste
• Grated Parmesan cheese (optional)

Instructions:

1. In a large skillet, heat the olive oil over medium heat. Add the minced garlic and cook for 1 minute, until fragrant.

2. Add the spiralized or julienned zucchini noodles to the skillet. Sauté for 3•5 minutes, until the zucchini is tender but still has some bite.

3. Stir in the diced tomatoes, chopped basil, tomato paste, and dried oregano. Season with salt and pepper.

4. Reduce the heat to low and let the sauce simmer for 5•7 minutes, allowing the flavors to meld.

5. Serve the zucchini noodles with the tomato basil sauce. Top with grated Parmesan cheese if desired.

This dish is a great option for the Galveston Diet and menopause for several reasons:

• Zucchini noodles are a low•carb, high•fiber alternative to traditional pasta.
• Tomatoes are a good source of the antioxidant lycopene.
• Fresh basil provides anti•inflammatory benefits.
• The dish is gluten•free, dairy•free (without the optional Parmesan), and plant•based.

The combination of the tender zucchini noodles and the flavorful tomato basil sauce makes for a satisfying and nutritious meal. It's a great way to incorporate more vegetables into your diet while enjoying a pasta•like dish.

113. Mediterranean Chicken Skewers with Yogurt Sauce

Ingredient:

For the Chicken Skewers:
• 1 lb boneless, skinless chicken breasts, cut into 1•inch cubes
• 1 red onion, cut into 1•inch pieces
• 1 red bell pepper, cut into 1•inch pieces
• 1 zucchini, cut into 1•inch pieces
• 2 tbsp olive oil
• 1 tbsp lemon juice
• 2 tsp dried oregano
• 1 tsp ground cumin
• Salt and pepper to taste

For the Yogurt Sauce:
• 1 cup plain Greek yogurt
• 1 tbsp lemon juice
• 1 clove garlic, minced
• 2 tbsp chopped fresh parsley
• Salt and pepper to taste

Instructions:

1. In a large bowl, combine the chicken cubes, onion, bell pepper, and zucchini. Drizzle with the olive oil and lemon juice, then sprinkle with the oregano, cumin, salt, and pepper. Toss to coat the ingredients evenly.

2. Thread the chicken and vegetables onto skewers, alternating the ingredients.

3. Preheat your grill or grill pan to medium•high heat. Grill the skewers for 12•15 minutes, turning occasionally, until the chicken is cooked through and the vegetables are tender.

4. In a small bowl, mix together the Greek yogurt, lemon juice, minced garlic, and chopped parsley. Season with salt and pepper.

5. Serve the grilled Mediterranean Chicken Skewers warm, with the yogurt sauce on the side for dipping.

The combination of the flavorful grilled chicken and vegetables, along with the cooling yogurt sauce, makes this a delicious and nutritious meal. Enjoy these Mediterranean Chicken Skewers as part of your Galveston Diet and menopause•friendly meal plan.

114. Roasted Brussels Sprouts with Pecans and Cranberries

Ingredient:

• 1 lb Brussels sprouts, trimmed and halved
• 2 tbsp olive oil
• 1/2 tsp salt
• 1/4 tsp black pepper
• 1/2 cup pecan halves
• 1/3 cup dried cranberries
• 1 tbsp balsamic glaze (optional)

Instructions:

1. Preheat your oven to 400°F.

2. In a large bowl, toss the trimmed and halved Brussels sprouts with the olive oil, salt, and pepper until well coated.

3. Spread the Brussels sprouts in a single layer on a baking sheet.

4. Roast the Brussels sprouts for 18•22 minutes, tossing halfway, until they are tender and lightly browned.

5. Remove the Brussels sprouts from the oven and transfer them back to the large bowl.

6. Add the pecan halves and dried cranberries to the bowl. Toss gently to combine.

7. Drizzle the balsamic glaze over the Brussels sprouts mixture, if desired. Serve the Roasted Brussels Sprouts with Pecans and Cranberries warm.

This dish is a great option for the Galveston Diet and menopause for several reasons:

• Brussels sprouts are a low•carb, high•fiber vegetable that is rich in vitamins, minerals, and antioxidants.
• Pecans provide healthy fats, protein, and fiber.
• Dried cranberries add a touch of sweetness and antioxidants.
• The dish is gluten•free, dairy•free, and vegan.

The combination of the roasted Brussels sprouts, crunchy pecans, and tart cranberries creates a flavorful and nutrient•dense side dish. The balsamic glaze adds a nice touch of sweetness and acidity.

115. Berry Spinach Salad with Grilled Chicken

Ingredient:

- 4 cups fresh spinach leaves
- 1 cup mixed berries (such as blueberries, raspberries, blackberries)
- 4 oz grilled chicken breast, sliced
- 2 tbsp olive oil
- 1 tbsp balsamic vinegar
- Salt and pepper to taste

Instructions:

1. In a large salad bowl, combine the spinach and mixed berries.

2. Top with the sliced grilled chicken.

3. In a small bowl, whisk together the olive oil and balsamic vinegar. Season with salt and pepper.

4. Drizzle the dressing over the salad and toss gently to coat.

This salad is a great option for the Galveston Diet during menopause. It's packed with nutrient•dense spinach, antioxidant•rich berries, and lean protein from the grilled chicken. The healthy fats from the olive oil also help support hormone balance. The balsamic vinegar provides a tangy flavor without added sugar. Enjoy this refreshing and satisfying salad as a main dish or side.

Thank you for joining us on this culinary journey through ***"The Galveston Diet Cookbook for Menopause: 110+ Recipes Nourishing for Balanced Hormones."*** As you have explored these pages, you've discovered the powerful connection between the foods you eat and your overall well-being during menopause.

Menopause is a natural and transformative phase of life, and the right nutrition can significantly impact how you feel and function. The recipes in this book are designed to support hormonal balance, reduce inflammation, and provide the nutrients your body needs to thrive. By incorporating these delicious and nourishing meals into your daily routine, you are taking a proactive step towards enhancing your health and embracing this stage of life with vitality and grace.

Key Takeaways:

- ***Hormonal Balance:*** The recipes in this cookbook focus on ingredients that help balance hormones naturally, such as phytoestrogen-rich foods, healthy fats, and high-quality proteins.

- ***Anti-Inflammatory Diet:*** By reducing inflammation through the inclusion of anti-inflammatory foods, you can alleviate many common menopausal symptoms and improve overall health.

- ***Weight Management:*** The Galveston Diet emphasizes nutrient-dense, low-carb meals that support healthy weight management, helping you feel your best.

- ***Sustained Energy:*** With a focus on balanced macronutrients and intermittent fasting, these recipes are designed to stabilize blood sugar levels and provide lasting energy throughout the day.

- ***Enhanced Mood and Well-Being:*** Proper nutrition plays a crucial role in mental health. The ingredients chosen for these recipes support a positive mood and mental clarity.

Moving Forward:

As you continue on your journey beyond this cookbook, remember that small, consistent changes can lead to significant improvements in your health and well-being. Listen to your body, be mindful of how different foods affect you, and embrace the process of nourishing yourself with wholesome, delicious meals.

Stay Connected:

We encourage you to stay connected with the principles of the Galveston Diet and to continue exploring new recipes and ways to support your health. Consider joining a community of like-minded individuals who share your commitment to thriving during menopause and beyond. Sharing your experiences, challenges, and successes can be incredibly empowering and motivating.

Final Thoughts:

Menopause is not an end but a new beginning—a time to focus on your health, wellness, and personal growth. By embracing the Galveston Diet and incorporating these 110+ nourishing recipes into your life, you are taking a positive and proactive approach to this significant phase.

Thank you for allowing us to be a part of your journey. Here's to a balanced, vibrant, and fulfilling life during menopause and beyond. May your kitchen be filled with joy, creativity, and the delicious aromas of meals that nourish both body and soul.

With warmest wishes,

9 798329 710731